D0552738

Contents

Preface		iv
Executive advisory panel		vi
1	Introduction	1
2	From whose perspective?	13
3	Lay involvement: the who, what, where, when, why and how of involving lay people in research	21
4	Lay involvement strategies	43
5	Vignettes from the literature	53
6	Wider issues in lay involvement	67
7	Research methods	77
8	Questions to ask before getting involved in research	97
9	Regulation of patient data: Caldicott Guardians	103
10	Research ethics committees	107
11	Human rights and ethics: guidelines and contacts	121
12	Successful marketing and public relations for your research project	125
Appendix 1: Additional sources of help and advice		129
Appendix 2: Contacts for various projects used in this text		137
Index		139

Preface

The primary purpose of this book is to provide some vignettes and guidance for healthcare professionals who are likely to be, or are already inclined, to have lay involvement in their health research. Such involvement is increasingly being supported and promoted by politicians, policy makers, funders, managers, healthcare professionals, advisory panels, consumer and lay advocates. There is also growing pressure from the media to get more lay involvement in health research.

Health research is now a multimillion pound business, with a variety of sources of funding, aims and objectives. Sources of funding include governments, their agents and agencies, pharmaceutical and other healthcare companies, insurance companies, not-for-profit organisations, charities, academic institutions, and dedicated research sponsors.

Health research is an international business. A considerable number of research studies have taken place and will continue to take place across nations, and studies that take place in one nation or set of nations may have application and relevance to other countries. There are also an increasing number of international standards, rules and regulations associated with health research.

Lay involvement in research is occurring in a wide variety of places, locally and beyond. Lay involvement is also on the increase in decision-making committees and boards, such as service planning, resource allocation and deployment. The bottom line is of course the focus on what you can do locally with your lay involvement that really matters.

Healthcare is not the first or only place to encourage lay involvement in research. This book provides some insights from other places. For example lay involvement currently takes place in social care, education, law and order, community development, transport, environment, finance and housing, to name a few areas, so the concept itself is not new. Therefore this book can be seen to offer general points, thoughts and lessons for lay involvement in research.

Even when rewarding, lay involvement is not an easy option, and you will come across some people who frown on the idea, others who have refused or will refuse to fund such involvement, and others still who dismiss research with such involvement as 'dumbing down' research and suggest it is somehow 'non-scientific'. From what I have seen and experienced I am confident enough to suggest that in a few years' time these types of people, their ideas and ideals, will become relatively more scarce, diluting their rather shocking and sanctimonious positions. The sceptics to lay involvement in health research should not be silenced, as their calls and concerns can only serve to whet the appetite for more genuine involvement and to encourage the building of strong banks of evidence of the merits and worth of lay involvement in health research.

Some research sponsors already make it a general rule that to apply for funding from them means you have to have lay involvement in the research plan. Local media can be gainfully used to help in all aspects of the research from running through ideas, to running the project, to recruitment, and results circulation. Further down the line, lay involvement can be gainfully used to aid the dissemination and uptake of research results.

How can you use this book? Here are some ideas.

- If you come across a concept that may be used in lay involvement in research and need clarification, refer to this book.
- When you want to learn some of the tools of the trade of lay involvement in research, refer to this book.
- When you want to use lay involvement ideas in your own work, check with this book to help you on your way.
- Use it to check for updates and announcements on lay involvement activities appearing on the web e.g. from the research councils, INVOLVE (the renamed Consumers in NHS Research Support Unit) (www.invo.org.uk), from pharmaceutical companies, governments, charities and other sponsors of quality research.
- Participate – if there is an issue in lay involvement in research that you think could be included in the next edition of this book, or if you have good examples you think a wider audience would appreciate very much, contact me (alaneslater@hotmail.com).

Many people helped to formulate this book and I wish to thank them for showing enthusiasm and commitment to sharing their experiences of lay involvement in research. Organisations that have kindly and generously helped are identified in the appendices.

A special thank-you goes to my executive advisory panel. They can take full credit for what they have done to improve this book, and I openly acknowledge their tact, diplomacy, understanding, inspiration and patience.

Executive advisory panel

- Professor Ann Bowling, Professor of Health Services Research, Department of Primary Care and Population Sciences, University College Medical School, London.
- Wendy Garlick, Principal Policy Advisor – Health, Consumers' Association, 2 Marylebone Road, London.
- Dr Warwick Hunt, Head of Clinical Governance and Quality Development, Northamptonshire Health Authority, Northampton.
- Ms Jane Neal, Director of Medicines Information, Pharmacy Department, Northwick Park NHS Hospital, Harrow.
- Professor Tom Walley, Department of Pharmacology and Therapeutics, University of Liverpool, Liverpool.

Chapter 1

Introduction

The primary purpose of this book is to provide some vignettes and guidance for healthcare professionals who are beginning to be inclined, or are already inclined, to have lay involvement in their health research.

Such involvement is increasingly being supported and promoted by politicians, policy makers, funders, managers, healthcare professionals, advisory panels, consumer and lay advocates. There is also growing pressure from the media to get more lay involvement in health research.

In August 2002 for example, the UK's National Institute for Clinical Excellence (NICE) announced it was setting up a 'Citizens Council'. The idea behind this is that the Citizens Council would help NICE find out what members of the public think about key issues that inform the development of guidance that NICE issues on the use of treatments and the care that people can receive in the NHS. The Citizens Council will consist of 30 people from a cross section of the community and meet twice a year for three consecutive days. NICE offers a short introduction to Citizens Councils, and guidance can be found on its website.[1] Members of the Citizens Council have been appointed for variable periods so that they do not all leave at the same time. Council members suggested they have more involvement in the calling of expert witnesses – something the NICE board agreed with.

The first meeting of the NICE Citizens Council took place in November 2002. At a public meeting in January 2003 NICE considered a list of recommendations from the Citizens Council. The Citizens Council had been asked to consider what NICE should and should not take into account in its appraisals of *clinical* need. The council said that NICE should not take into account the social and economic circumstances of patients, should not take into account whether the diseases or conditions were 'self-inflicted', and should not take into account how 'loud' the voice of the patient was/is. Many questions remain for following through the implications of these ideas (e.g. think of a smoker needing a heart transplant, an obese patient needing a hip replacement).

In terms of the members of the Citizens Council, some issues remain – for instance the lack of young and old people serving on the council compared to the number of young and old people under NHS care. The ethnic mix may also need careful attention and the council needs to give due attention in its recruitment so that the disenfranchised and marginalised in our society have a voice. Finally, whether the NICE Citizens Council calls for more lay involvement in research and for more lay involvement in the research work that NICE bases its decisions on remains to be seen.

In 2002 the Department of Health and Social Care Research and Development Office of London funded 11 primary care projects on issues such as a lay-led self-management programme with chronic illness in Bengalis, promoting testicular self-examination and awareness among young men with learning disabilities. Active consumer involvement was a condition of funding. As important, it set aside funding for training and development support and for two assessments of the impact of that training and development.

Earlier in the summer of 2002, the Medical Research Council (MRC), a publicly-funded sponsor of medical research in the UK, began conducting a major review of its approach to supporting clinical research. The closing date for submitting a contribution to the review was 31 August 2002. The reasons for the review, which included taking evidence and opinions from a variety of stakeholders, are that the demand for objective evidence to underpin and drive changes in clinical practice is greater than ever before; trials are becoming larger, often multicentre international ventures; the pace of change means new ideas, products and techniques are becoming superseded relatively quicker than ever before; evidence must be generated quickly; people's expectations are growing; accountability procedures are being made more transparent; and regulations around the whole business of research are changing. Amongst the questions the MRC sought views on were the opportunities for the MRC to work more closely with 'consumer groups', how consumers should be involved in the different stages of the trial process and how consumers find out about trials. The word 'consumer' is largely undefined by the MRC.

In late 2002 the BUPA Foundation offered funding of up to £500 000 to advance thinking and practice on innovative and critical projects that address consumer involvement in healthcare, particularly where the involvement ensures better outcomes with available resources.

Lay involvement currently takes place in social care, education, law and order, community development, transport, environment, finance, and housing to name a few areas, so the concept itself is not new.

Even when rewarding, lay involvement is not an easy option, and I have no doubt that you will come across some people who frown on the idea, others who have refused or will refuse to fund involvement, and others still who dismiss research with such involvement as 'dumbing down' research and 'non-scientific'. I am confident enough to suggest that in a few years time these types of people, their ideas and ideals, will become relatively scarce rather than shocking and sanctimonious. Yet they should not be silenced, as their calls and concerns can only serve to whet the appetite for more genuine involvement and to encourage the building of strong banks of evidence of the merits and worth of lay involvement in health research.

What motivated me to write this book was to provide some sort of guide to colleagues in health who are thinking about having, or already have, lay involvement in healthcare research. But before I wrote the master plan for this piece of work I quickly realised that much of what I was about to say has relevance to another audience: all those lay people that may become involved in health research. Therefore, as I planned and penned away, I was very conscious that this book should be of some value to lay people who may get involved in health research projects and programmes.

Following this introductory chapter, I then move on to outline some issues in terms of perspectives in healthcare. Chapter 3 provides a sketch of a variety of issues such as the rationale for lay involvement in research, who to involve, what they can do, where they can be involved, where to find lay people, how they can be involved, when to have lay involvement, and payment for lay members. Chapter 4 looks at lay involvement strategies, and what makes for successful lay involvement. Vignettes from the literature are outlined in Chapter 5, with Chapter 6 taking a glimpse at wider issues of lay involvement. Chapter 7 describes research methods employed in projects with lay members, which is then followed by a chapter on questions to ask before getting involved in a research project. Chapters 9, 10, and 11 provide insight and contacts for the regulation of patient data, ethics committee work and human rights. The final chapter is about the tools, tips and traps of marketing and public relations exercises for your research project. The appendices provide contact information on sources of help and advice.

In addition to this book, lay involvement groups themselves will have experience and expertise in their own particular fields upon which you may, indeed should, be able to call. The more you get insight from other parties, the more likely you are to become equipped to effectively and efficiently include lay involvement in your research.

A word about terminology is warranted. 'Lay involvement' means different things to different people: there is no one fixed universally acceptable definition. Lay involvement in healthcare research means to me anyone who is not a healthcare professional or current patient on the topic getting involved, or being involved, in structured research on that topic. Lay members could for instance be past patients, non-patients, their friends and family (*see* Figure 1.1). There are various ethical, practical, logistical, legal and moral issues when a current patient as a *subject* of the research (i.e. under investigation) is also a *member* of the research team (i.e. part of the investigating team). This is why I suggest the terms 'past patients' and 'non-patients' in Figure 1.1.

In general by lay involvement I mean a person who is not and never has been:

- a doctor, dentist, ophthalmic medical practitioner, optician or pharmacist
- a registered dispensing optician
- a registered nurse, registered midwife or registered health visitor
- an officer of, or someone otherwise employed by any health board, health authority, local health council, patient forum (excluding community health councils) or primary care trust.

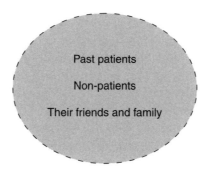

Figure 1.1: Lay people.

By the term involvement I use the following definition: 'the involvement of lay members in the research, rather than being the recipients or the subjects of the product or service under study'.

There will, in reality, be exceptions to this, but it is the preferred definition. Other terms and definitions that have been used include consumers, customers, stakeholders, partners, citizens, clients and service users. These descriptors may be quite meaningful to some but they have had different meanings in different contexts. If you feel more comfortable with any of these terms, use them.

But as a note of caution, there is fresh evidence that the word 'consumer' has various unpalatable connotations. For example Telford and colleagues[2] provide recent evidence that the word 'consumer':

- implies the doctor is running a supermarket
- sits with the language of buying and selling, and seems inappropriate for the types of relationships which exist in a health service

- implies they themselves consume the products or services under study
- suggests that they have a choice, when in fact many do not.

Table 1.1 provides an indication of current examples of lay involvement. These examples will be discussed in more detail throughout the book.

Table 1.1: Current examples of lay involvement

Title of topic	Aims of project
Cancer voices	To explore ways in which cancer service users can get their voices heard in cancer services and research
Patient and carer views of stroke services	To identify patient and carer recommendations of topics/issues to be addressed by a national clinical guideline
A randomised controlled trial to evaluate the benefit of a new information leaflet for parents of children hospitalised with benign febrile convulsions	To test the impact of the leaflet in terms of parents' understanding and behavioural knowledge of febrile convulsions. To assess changes in parents' anxiety levels following discharge and parents' satisfaction with the discharge information provided
A large randomised long-term assessment of the relative cost-effectiveness of surgery for Parkinson's disease	To evaluate the cost-effectiveness of subthalmic nucleus surgery and also the timing of surgery, compared with active medical therapy
Survey of views of people affected by motor neurone disease on the only drug treatment (then) available: riluzole	To assimilate the views of people affected by motor neurone disease in order to inform the Motor Neurone Disease Association's submission to NICE
Evaluating the multiple sclerosis (MS) specialist nurse: a review and development of the role	To identify and describe the employment patterns, profile and views of MS nurses about their role in the UK. To look for evidence of one nurse's contribution to care for people with MS in West Berkshire, taking into account the views of local stakeholders relating to reviewing and developing the service
Torbay Healthy Housing Group: Watcombe Project	To assess the extent to which housing conditions affect the indoor environment, health (particularly respiratory health) and wellbeing of residents, and the cost to the NHS
Medication education	To evaluate the usefulness of medication education for patients on an intensive care ward
Befriending: more than just finding friends?	To understand different models of befriending. To evaluate befriending services. To analyse factors that prevent people being able to access befriending services
Practice guidelines for primary healthcare teams to meet South Asian carers' needs	To explore the experiences and needs of South Asian carers and their encounters with primary healthcare services. To elicit their views about how primary healthcare services could support them. To develop a set of practical guidelines for use by primary care teams, based on the findings of the first two objectives

Table 1.1: Continued

Title of topic	Aims of project
What happens to people with severe aphasia?	To find out about the experience of severe aphasia (language impairment) through: a national survey of therapists and voluntary associations; in-depth ethnographic study of 20 people with severe aphasia
Collaborative studies on health service and quality of life in people with learning disability	To improve the quality of life and promote social inclusion for people with learning disability
Joint replacement	To understand the barriers to appropriate utilisation of joint replacements and to test alternatives
Cognitive remediation: a randomised controlled trial	To evaluate the success of cognitive remediation therapy in improving cognition, social functioning and self-esteem
People's experiences of screening assessment by nurses in a community mental health team	To develop theory which will assist the understanding of the processes affecting involvement in mental health screening assessment
Disability equipment evaluations	To gather information from users and carers about how disability products meet their needs. To compile guidelines to assist appropriate choice of product
Cochrane skin group	To conduct a systematic review of existing research (randomised controlled trials). To establish the efficacy of medical interventions
Developing and evaluating best practice for user involvement in cancer services	The project is looking at user involvement in the planning, delivery and evaluation of cancer services. The aim is to identify effective and appropriate ways of involving users and to develop a way of monitoring and evaluating user involvement in cancer services

References

1 National Institute for Clinical Excellence (NICE) (2002) *UK's first Citizens Council being established by NICE*. NICE, London.
2 Telford R, Beverley CA, Cooper CL et al. (2002) Consumer involvement in health research: fact or fiction? *Br J Clin Gov*. **7**: 92–103.

Further reading

• Aman MG and Wolford PL (1995) Consumer satisfaction with involvement in drug research: a social validity study. *J Am Acad Child Adolesc Psychiatry*. **34**: 940–5.

- Arnstein SR (1969) A ladder of citizen participation. *Journal of American Institute of Planners.* **35**(4): 216–61.
- Barnes M and Wistow G (eds) (1992) *Researching User Involvement.* The Nuffield Institute for Health Services Seminar Series, University of Leeds, Leeds.
- Bastian H (1996) Raising the standard: practice guidelines and consumer participation. *Int J Qual Health Care.* **8**: 485–90.
- Bastian H (1994) *The Power of Sharing Knowledge: consumer participation in the Cochrane Collaboration.* Cochrane Collaboration Consumer Network, December.
- Baxter L, Thorne L and Mitchell A (undated) *Small Voices: big noises: lay involvement in health research: lessons from other fields.* Folk.us Programme, University of Exeter, Exeter.
- Beresford P (undated) Researching citizen-involvement: a collaborative or colonising enterprise? In: Barnes M and Wistow G *Researching User Involvement.* The Nuffield Institute for Health Services Studies, University of Leeds.
- Boote J, Telford R and Cooper C (2002) Consumer involvement in health research: a review and research agenda. *Health Policy.* **61**: 213–36.
- Chalmers I (1994) *Public involvement in research to assess the effects of healthcare.* Paper to the Harveian Society of London. UK Cochrane Centre, Oxford.
- Consumers in NHS Research (1998) *Research: what's in it for consumers?* Standing Advisory Group on Consumer Involvement in the NHS R&D Programme. Department of Health, London.
- Consumers in NHS Research (2000) *Involving Consumers in Randomised Controlled Trials.* Seminar report. CNHSR Support Unit Eastleigh, Hampshire.
- Consumers in NHS Research (2000) *Involving Consumers in Commissioning Health Research.* Seminar report. CNHSR Support Unit Eastleigh, Hampshire.
- Consumers in NHS Research (2001) *Involving consumers? An exploration of consumer involvement in NHS R&D managed by Department of Health Regional Offices.* CNHSR Support Unit Eastleigh, Hampshire.
- Consumers in NHS Research (2002) *Involving Consumers. Briefing notes for researchers.* CNHSR Support Unit Eastleigh, Hampshire.
- Coats AJ (2000) Consumer involvement in cardiovascular research: ways to combat bias and secrecy. *Int J Cardiol.* **75**: 1–3.
- Congressionally Directed Medical Research Programs (CDMRP) (1998) Perspective from the Department of Defense Breast Cancer Research Program. *Breast Disease.* **10**: 33–45.
- Congressionally Directed Medical Research Programs (2002) *How can other organizations set up a program to involve consumers?* CDMRP, Maryland, USA.
- Consumers' Health Forum of Australia (1990) *Guidelines for Consumer Representatives: suggestions for consumer or community representatives*

working on public committees. Consumers' Health Forum of Australia, Canberra.

- Davies C (2001) *Lay involvement in professional regulation.* School of Health and Social Welfare, The Open University, Buckingham.
- Department of Health (1999) *Patient and Public Involvement in the New NHS.* Department of Health, London.
- Department of Health (2000) *Working Partnerships 3rd Report.* Department of Health, London.
- Department of Health (2001) *Involving Patients and the Public in Healthcare: a discussion document.* Department of Health, London.
- Department of Health (2002) *Consumer Involvement: consumers in NHS research.* Department of Health, London.
- Department of Health (2002) *Research and Development in the NHS: an introductory guide.* Department of Health, London.
- Dixon P, Peart E and Carr-Hill R (1999) *A Database and Report on Consumer Involvement in Research.* University of York, York.
- Domenighetti G (1994) From ethics of ignorance to consumers empowerment. *Soc Prev Med.* **39**: 123–5.
- Dwyer J (1989) The politics of participation. *Comm Health Studies.* **13**: 59–65.
- Earl-Slater A (2002) *The Handbook of Clinical Trials and other Research.* Radcliffe Medical Press, Oxford.
- Entwistle V, Renfrew M, Yearly S *et al.* (1998) Lay perspectives: advantages for health research. *BMJ.* **316**: 463–6.
- Entwistle VA, Sheldon TA, Sowden AJ *et al.* (1996) Supporting consumer involvement in decision making: what constitutes quality in consumer health information? *Int J Qual Health Care.* **8**: 425–37.
- Evans C and Fisher M (1999) Collaborative evaluation with service users: moving towards user-controlled research. In: Shaw I and Lishman J (eds) *Evaluation in Social Work.* Sage Publications, London.
- Faulkner A and Thomas P (2002) User-led research and evidence-based medicine. *Br J Psychiatry.* **180**: 1–3.
- Fleming B and Golding L (1997) *Involving Users* vol. 1. Soundings Research, Birmingham.
- Flower J and Wirz S (2000) Rhetoric or reality? The participation of disabled people in NGO planning. *Health Policy Plan.* **15**: 177–85.
- Flynn BC, Wiles DW and Rider MS (1994) Empowering communities: action research through healthy cities. *Health Educ Q.* **21**: 395–405.
- Gann B (1994) *Making decisions in the year 2000: realising the potential of consumer health information services.* Fourth European Conference for Medical and Health Care Libraries, Oslo.
- Goodare H and Lockwood S (1999) Involving patients in clinical research: improves the quality of research. *BMJ.* **319**: 724–5.
- Goodare H and Smith R (1995) The rights of patients in research. *BMJ.* **310**: 1277–8.

- Hamilton-Gurney B (1994) *Public Participation in Health Care. Involving the public in healthcare decision making: a critical review of the issues and methods.* East Anglian Regional Health Authority, Cambridge.
- Hanley B, on behalf of the Standing Group on Consumers in NHS Research (1999) *Involvement Works: the second report of the Standing Group on Consumers in NHS Research.* Department of Health, London.
- Hanley B (1999) Research and development in the NHS: how can you make a difference? *Health Expect.* **2**: 72.
- Hares T, Spencer J, Gallagher M *et al.* (1992) Diabetes care: who are the experts? *Q Health Care.* **1**: 219–24.
- Heller T, Pederson EL and Miller AB (1996) Guidelines from the consumer: improving consumer involvement in research and training for persons with mental retardation. *Ment Retard.* **34**: 141–8.
- Help for Health Trust (undated) *Training for Professionals, Lay Representatives and Consumers.* The Help for Health Trust, Winchester, Hampshire.
- Herxheimer A (1988) The rights of the patient in clinical research. *Lancet.* **2**(8620): 1128–30.
- Hogg C (1999) *Patients, Power and Politics.* Sage Publications, London.
- House of Lords Select Committee on Science and Technology (1995) *Medical Research and the NHS Reforms.* HL Paper 12, Session 1994–95, 3rd report. HMSO, London.
- House of Lords Select Committee on Science and Technology (1988) *Priorities in Medical Research* vol. 1 – report. HMSO, London.
- Irwin A (1995) *Citizen science: a study of people, expertise and sustainable development.* Routledge, London.
- Jakubowska D and Crossley P (1999) Developing skills in consulting with the public. *BMJ.* **319**: 2–3.
- Johnson M (undated) *The Involvement of Black and Minority Ethnic Consumers in Health Research and Development: a report to accompany the SAGCI database.* University of Warwick.
- Kelson M (1998) *Promoting Consumer Involvement in Clinical Audit: practical guidelines on achieving effective involvement.* College of Health, London.
- Kelson M (1997) *User Involvement: a guide to developing effective user involvement strategies in the NHS.* College of Health, London.
- Khunti K (1999) Use of multiple methods to determine factors affecting quality of care of patients with diabetes. *Fam Pract.* **16**: 489–94.
- Liberati A (1997) Consumer participation in research and healthcare: making it a reality. *BMJ.* **315**: 499.
- Local Management Government Board (1994) *Community participation in local agenda 21.* Local Government Management Board (local agenda 21 round table guidance), Luton.
- Macaulay AC, Commanda LE, Freeman WL *et al.* (1999) Participatory research maximises community and lay involvement. *BMJ.* **319**: 774–8.

- Matrice D and Brown V (eds) (1990) *Widening the Research Focus: consumer roles in public health research.* Consumers' Health Forum of Australia, Canberra.
- McNeill PM, Berglund CA and Webster IW (1994) How much influence do various members have within research ethics committees? *Camb Q Healthc Ethics.* Special Section: Research Ethics. **3**: 522–32.
- Morris J (undated) *Don't Leave Us Out: involving disabled children and young people with communication impairment.* York Publishing Services, York.
- Morris J (1996) *Encouraging user involvement in commissioning: a resource for commissioners.* NHS Executive/Department of Health, Leeds.
- National Coordinating Centre for Health Technology Assessment (1999) *Annual Report of the NHS Health Technology Assessment Programme 1998.* Department of Health, London.
- National Institute for Clinical Excellence (NICE) (2002) *A Short Introduction to the Citizens Council.* NICE, London.
- National Institute for Clinical Excellence (NICE) (2002) *Common Questions and Answers on the Citizens Council.* NICE, London.
- National Consumer Council (2003) *Stronger Voice – training resources.* National Consumer Council, London.
- Neuberger J (1999) Let's do away with 'patients'. *BMJ.* **318**: 1756–7.
- Newell C (1992) Consumer participation in the bioethics of disability. *Health Forum.* **22**: 11–13.
- NHS Executive (1999) *Involvement Works* 2nd report. NHS Executive, Leeds.
- NHS Executive (1998) *Research: What's in it for Consumers?* 1st report. NHS Executive, Leeds.
- North West Regional R&D Office (2002) *Making it Happen: action planning for user involvement in R&D* (a report of an action research workshop held in April 2001). R&D Directorate, North West Regional R&D Office, Warrington.
- North West Regional R&D Office (2002) *User Involvement in NHS Provider Organisations* (a report of trusts in receipt of support funding). R&D Directorate, North West Regional R&D Office, Warrington.
- Ochocka J, Janzen R and Nelson G (2002) Sharing power and knowledge: professional and mental health consumer/survivor researchers working together in a participatory action research project. *Psychiatr Rehabil J.* **25**: 379–87.
- Office of Science and Technology and the Wellcome Trust (2000) *Science and the Public: a review of science communication and public attitudes to science in Britain.* DTI and Wellcome Trust, London.
- Oliver S (1996) The progress of lay involvement in the NHS Research and Development Programme. *J Eval Clin Pract.* **2**: 273–80.
- Oliver SR (1995) How can health service users contribute to the NHS research and development programme? *BMJ.* **310**: 1318–20.

- Ong BN (1996) The lay perspective in health technology assessment. *Int J Technol Assess Health Care.* **12**: 511–17.
- Pfeffer N (1994) Creating dialogues: community health councils. In: Dunning M and Needham G (eds) *But Will It Work, Doctor?* Report of a conference about involving users of health services in outcomes research. The Consumer Health Information Consortium, UK.
- Royle J, Steel R, Hanley B *et al.* (undated) *Getting Involved in Research: a guide for consumers.* Consumers in NHS Research Support Unit Eastleigh, Hampshire.
- Russell H and Szoke H (1990) *Review of Consumer Participation in the National Health and Medical Research Council.* Consumers' Health Forum of Australia, Canberra.
- Schwarcz SL (moderator) (1981) Non-scientist participation in the peer review process: Is it desirable? Is it implementable? Who are the non-scientists who should become involved? A panel discussion. *Ann NY Academy Sci.* **2**: 213–28.
- Sheppard B (2002) *Making a Start: involving older people in the doctor's surgery.* Age Concern, London.
- Simeonsson RJ, Edmondson R, Smith T *et al.* (1995) Family involvement in multidisciplinary team evaluation: professional and parent perspectives. *Child Care Health Dev.* **21**: 199–214 (comment 214–15).
- Simpson E, House AO and Barkham M (2002) *A Guide to Involving Users, Ex-users and Carers in Mental Health Service Planning, Delivery and Research: a health technology approach.* University of Leeds, Leeds.
- Standing Group on Consumers in NHS Research (1999) *Strategic Alliances Workshop 27 January 1999: workshop report.* Help for Health Trust, Winchester.
- Tallon D, Chard J and Dieppe P (2000) Consumer involvement in research is essential. *BMJ.* **320**: 380–1.
- Telford R (2002) *Successful Consumer Involvement in Research: an evaluation using consensus-generated criteria.* School of Health and Related Research, Sheffield.
- Thorne L, Putsell R and Baxter L (2001) *Knowing How – a guide to getting involved in research.* Folk.us, Exeter University CNHSR, Exeter.
- Thornton H (1998) Alliance between medical profession and consumers already exists in breast cancer. *BMJ.* **316**: 148–9.
- Thornton H (1995) *The Patient's Role in Research.* In: Health Committee, Third Report vol. II. HMSO, London.
- Tighe RJ and Biersdorff KK (1993) Setting agendas for relevant research: a participatory approach. *Can J Rehab.* **7**: 127–32.
- Truman C and Raine P (2002) Experience and meaning of user involvement: some explorations from a community mental health project. *Health Soc Care Community.* **10**: 136–43.
- US Department of the Army (1998) *Congressionally Directed Medical Research Programs, Fiscal Year 1998. Status report.* Fort Detrick, MD, US Army Medical Research and Material Command.

- Wadsworth Y (1990) The consumer contribution to public health research and its funding administration. In: Matrice D and Brown V (eds) *Widening the Research Focus: consumer roles in public health research.* Consumers' Health Forum of Australia, Canberra.
- Williamson C (1999) Medical research needs lay involvement. *J Med Ethics.* **25**: 62.
- Williamson C (2001) What does involving consumers in research mean? *Q J Med.* **94**: 661–4.
- World Health Organization (1978) *Declaration of Alma Ata: report of the International Conference on Primary Health Care.* WHO, Geneva.
- Yearley S (1994) Understanding science from the perspective of the sociology of scientific knowledge: an overview. *Public Underst Sci.* **3**: 245–58.
- Yelding D (1992) *Consumers and Health.* A report for the Consumer Policy Service, by the Research Institute for Consumer Affairs, UK.

Chapter 2

From whose perspective?

Thousands of research studies, costing millions of pounds, involving a large number of people are, at any moment in time, taking place. How many of them have involved lay people in their design, execution or interpretation? What are the costs and benefits of lay involvement in such aspects of health research? More fundamentally, how should lay involvement become embedded in such research? How can you get and maintain lay members' active involvement? Who should you involve? What are the ethics, logistics and practical problems of having consumer involvement in clinical research?

The perspective refers to the viewpoint adopted in an analysis. Matters very soon become very complicated because lay people come from different areas and any one may indeed have a different viewpoint from another. So rather than think of lay representativeness in your research team, think of taking lay people as being able to offer lay perspectives. If you want more than one lay perspective you will need to include more than one lay person. There are other perspectives in healthcare to consider and Figure 2.1 gives an overview.

While all these perspectives may have some common ground, e.g. they all want more effective and more efficient research and more compassionate healthcare, their particular perspectives on any issue can differ. Indeed there is evidence that their viewpoint depends on their place and time – e.g. if a patient has the disease their viewpoint may differ to views they held earlier; if a consultant wants to expand their service based on a new drug then their view, and that of others, will change as opportunities to diagnose and treat change.

Viewpoints also differ amongst groups of people. For example, Wellwood and colleagues[1] found that for patients with inguinal hernias, patients preferred laparoscopic rather than open-mesh hernia repair although the former was more expensive. Other parties may not believe the extra cost is worth it.

In an assessment of family involvement in multidisciplinary team evaluation of special education, Simeonsson and colleagues[2] used survey data from 39 parents and 81 professionals and found substantial

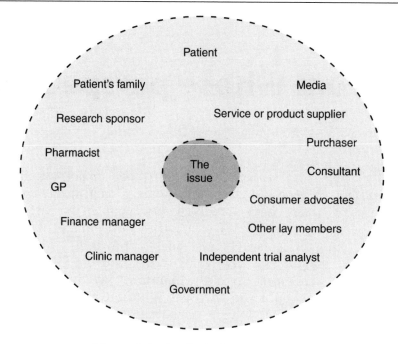

Figure 2.1: Analytical perspectives.

variability of perceptions among parents and professionals about the nature of child assessment and their respective roles in it.

Montgomery and Fahey[3] sought to explore how closely patients and clinicians agree in their preferences for different treatment options. Only studies that made quantifiable estimates of preferences were included. Montgomery and Fahey[3] found there is some evidence that patients and health professionals often do not agree on treatment preference in the areas of cardiovascular disease, cancer, obstetrics and gynaecology, and acute respiratory illness. To complicate matters, but to make them more realistic, Montgomery and Fahey[3] found that the magnitude and direction of these differences vary and may depend on the level of interest.

Probably some of the first real slivers of light have now been shed on perspectives and experiences of involving lay members in designing, conducting and interpreting randomised controlled trials. Hanley and colleagues[4] reported on a national study of clinical trial co-ordinating centres in the UK to assess the extent to which lay people were involved in the work of clinical trial co-ordinating centres and the nature of lay people's involvement in randomised trials co-ordinated by these centres.

Positive comments are reproduced in Box 2.1.

Box 2.1: Positive comments from investigators about involving lay people in trials

- **Setting the scene**
  - They were important in helping to refine the questions.
  - More relevant and clearer questions were asked.
  - They pushed hard for the trial.
  - They helped convince researchers and funders that the trial was possible and ethical.
  - They were useful in developing patient-centred outcome measures.
  - They provided important insights into how to make the trial work.
- **Informing participants**
  - They were important in helping refine information.
  - They helped make a complex trial comprehensible to most patients.
  - The backing and input of the range of relevant consumer groups undoubtedly improved the quality of information given to potential participants.
  - They had an impact on the type of information given about the trial: the leaflet was produced to fully inform patients about risks associated with their treatment.
  - They were able to increase their knowledge of the rationale for the trial.
- **Recruiting participants**
  - They provided insights into issues important to the community and patients.
  - Their participation led to improved recruitment.
  - They played a pivotal role in providing 'front line' intelligence on how the trial was being received during its development and execution.
- **Advocating for the trial**
  - A similar US trial was stopped prematurely and they felt it important to continue with the trial.
- **Disseminating information**
  - They provided a link to networks which helped publicise the trial.
- **Owning the trial**
  - They brought a sense of ownership of the concept and design of the trial to all who were involved and affected.
  - They helped build relationships that have enabled more proactive involvement in a trial that followed on from a particular study.

Box 2.2 provides another set of comments from investigators about involvement in trials. Hanley and colleagues[4] called them 'negative comments' but I see them as additional insights, learning points, into improving lay involvement in health research.

Box 2.2: Other comments from investigators about lay involvement in trials

- There need to be clear guidelines as to their remit so expectations are not disappointed.
- The problem is that there is no such thing as a 'representative': they are individuals often with totally conflicting viewpoints. Also their knowledge and understanding of trials vary greatly.
- At the moment there is no obvious impact.
- Their role in this particular project was not great.
- The whole process took much longer.
- The involvement of the community health council somewhat jeopardised the usefulness of the data. Their insistence that patients should not be sent a reminder letter resulted in a low response rate and poor representativeness of our sample.

While the evidence from Hanley and colleagues[4] relates to investigators' comments from involvement in specific clinical trials, there is no reason to believe that involvement would not be beneficial in any type of research, clinical trial or otherwise. In fact should sponsors of research, including the government spending taxpayers' money, their agents, charities, research foundations, health technology manufacturers and pharmaceutical companies now mandate that consumer involvement must be in all the research they fund hereinafter? If so how? If not, why not?

The bottom line is that people's perspectives vary (and can change over time or with different information before them) and therefore preferences need to be made more explicit when thinking of having lay involvement in your research. The challenge is to map and trace out these perspectives.

References

1 Wellwood J, Sculpher MJ, Stoker D et al. (1998) Randomised controlled trial of laparoscopic versus open mesh repair for inguinal hernia: outcome and cost. *BMJ.* **317**: 103–10.

2 Simeonsson RJ, Edmondson R, Smith T *et al.* (1995) Family involvement in multidisciplinary team evaluation: professional and parent perspectives. *Child Care Health Dev.* **21**: 199–214 (comment 214–15).

3 Montgomery AA and Fahey T (2001) How do patients' treatment preferences compare with those of clinicians? *Qual Health Care.* Suppl. **1**: 39–43.

4 Hanley B, Trusdale A, King A *et al.* (2001) Involving consumers in designing, conducting and interpreting randomised controlled trials: questionnaire survey. *BMJ.* **322**: 519–23.

Further reading

- Altman DG (1994) The scandal of poor medical research. *BMJ.* **308**: 283–4.
- Aman MG and Wolford PL (1995) Consumer satisfaction with involvement in drug research: a social validity study. *J Am Acad Child Adolesc Psychiatry.* **34**: 940–5.
- Andejeski Y, Bisceglio IT, Dickersin K *et al.* (2002) Quantitative impact of including consumers in the scientific review of breast cancer research proposals. *J Womens Health Gend Based Med.* **11**: 379–88.
- Bastian H (1994) *The Power of Sharing Knowledge: consumer participation in the Cochrane Collaboration.* Cochrane Collaboration Consumer Network, December.
- Bell RW, Damrosch SP and Lenz ER (1994) The polio survivor as expert: implications for nursing rehabilitation research. *Rehab Nurs.* **19**: 198–202.
- Bradburn J, Maher J, Adewuyi-Dalton R *et al.* (1995) Developing clinical trial protocols; the use of patient focus groups. *Psycho-Oncology.* **4**: 107–12.
- Campbell M, Entwistle V, Langston A *et al.* (2002) Scoping study to explore the most appropriate way to produce and disseminate information on randomised control trials. Health Services Research Unit, University of Aberdeen.
- Center for Communication Dynamics (1992) *Attitudes of Advocacy Groups: AIDS and cancer policy.* Rhone-Poulenc Rorer Inc., Pennsylvania.
- Chalmers I (2000) A guide to patient-led good controlled trials. *Lancet.* **356**: 774.
- Coats AJ (2000) Consumer involvement in cardiovascular research: ways to combat bias and secrecy. *Int J Cardiol.* **75**: 1–3.
- Congressionally Directed Medical Research Programs (CDMRP) (1998) Perspective from the Department of Defense Breast Cancer Research Program. *Breast Disease.* **10**: 33–45.
- Congressionally Directed Medical Research Programs (CDMRP) (2002) *How Can Other Organizations Set Up a Program to Involve Consumers?* Congressionally Directed Medical Research Programs, Maryland, USA.
- Coulter A, Peto V and Doll H (1994) Patients' preferences and general practitioners' decisions in the treatment of menstrual disorders. *Family Pract.* **11**: 67–74.

- Dixon P, Peart E and Carr-Hill R (1999) *A Database and Report on Consumer Involvement in Research*. University of York, York.
- Dolan JG, Bordley DR and Miller H (1993) Diagnostic strategies in the management of acute upper gastrointestinal bleeding: patient and physician preferences. *J Gen Intern Med*. **8**: 525–9.
- Drew NC, Salmon P and Webb I (1989) Mothers', midwives' and obstetricians' views on the features of obstetric care which influence satisfaction with childbirth. *Br J Obstet Gynaecol*. **96**: 1084–8.
- Earl-Slater A (2002) *The Handbook of Clinical Trials and Other Research*. Radcliffe Medical Press, Oxford.
- Ashcroft R (2000) Editorial. Giving medicine a fair trial. *BMJ*. **320**: 1686.
- Edwards SJL, Lilford RJ and Hewison J (1998) The ethics of randomised controlled trials from the perspectives of patients, the public, and healthcare professionals. *BMJ*. **317**: 1209–12.
- Entwistle V, Renfrew M, Yearly S *et al.* (1998) Lay perspectives: advantages for health research. *BMJ*. **316**: 463–6.
- Faulkner A and Thomas P (2002) User-led research and evidence-based medicine. *Br J Psychiatry*. **180**: 1–3.
- Featherstone K and Donovan JL (1998) Random allocation or allocation at random? Patients' perspectives of participation in a randomised controlled trial. *BMJ*. **317**: 1177–80.
- Flanagan J (1999) Public participation in the design of educational programmes for cancer nurses: a case report. *Eur J Cancer Care*. **8**: 107–12.
- Flower J and Wirz S (2000) Rhetoric or reality? The participation of disabled people in NGO planning. *Health Policy Plan*. **15**: 177–85.
- General Medical Council (1999) *Seeking Patients' Consent: the ethical considerations*. General Medical Council, London.
- Goodare H (ed) (1996) *Fighting Spirit: the stories of the women in the Bristol breast cancer survey*. Scarlet Press, London.
- Goodare H and Smith R (1995) The rights of patients in research. *BMJ*. **310**: 1277–8.
- Grol R, Weinman J, Dale J *et al.* (1999) Patient's priorities with respect to general practice care: an international comparison. *Fam Pract*. **16**: 4–11.
- Groome PA, Hutchinson TA and Tousignant P (1994) Content of a decision analysis for treatment choice in end stage renal disease: who should be consulted? *Br J Gen Pract*. **14**: 91–7.
- Hanley B (1999) *Involvement Works*. Department of Health, London.
- Hares T, Spencer J, Gallagher M *et al.* (1992) Diabetes care: who are the experts? *Q Health Care*. **1**: 219–24.
- Herxheimer A and Goodare H (1999) Who are you, and who are we? Looking through some key words. *Health Expect*. **2**: 3–6.
- Irwin A (1995) *Citizen Science: a study of people, expertise and sustainable development*. Routledge, London.
- Kelson M (1998) *Promoting Consumer Involvement in Clinical Audit: practical guidelines on achieving effective involvement*. College of Health, London.

- Khunti K (1999) Use of multiple methods to determine factors affecting quality of care of patients with diabetes. *Fam Pract.* **16**: 489–94.
- Klein S, Tracy D, Kitchener HC *et al.* (2000) The effects of participation of patients with cancer in teaching communication skills to medical undergraduates: a randomised study with follow-up after 2 years. *Eur J Cancer.* **36**: 273–81.
- Lee SK, Penner PL and Cox M (1991) Comparison of the attitudes of healthcare professionals and parents towards active treatment of very low birth weight infants. *Pediatrics.* **88**: 110–14.
- MacIlwain C (1993) AIDS activists say basic research is underfunded. *Nature.* **363**: 388.
- Marshall E (1993) The politics of breast cancer. *Science.* **259**: 616–17.
- McNeill PM, Berglund CA and Webster IW (1994) How much influence do various members have within research ethics committees? *Camb Q Healthc Ethics.* Special Section: Research Ethics **3**: 522–32.
- Morris J (undated) *Don't Leave Us Out: involving disabled children and young people with communication impairment.* York Publishing Services, York.
- Murray SA (1999) Experiences with 'rapid appraisal' in primary care: involving the public in assessing health needs, orientating staff, and educating medical students. *BMJ.* **318**: 440–4.
- National Institute for Clinical Excellence (NICE) (2002) *A Short Introduction to the Citizens Council.* NICE, London.
- Newell C (1992) Consumer participation in the bioethics of disability. *Health Forum.* **22**: 11–13.
- NHS Executive (1998) *Research: what's in it for consumers?* NHS Executive/ Department of Health, London.
- Nowak R (1995) AIDS researchers, activists, fight crisis in clinical trials. *Science.* **269**: 1666–7.
- Ochocka J, Janzen R and Nelson G (2002) Sharing power and knowledge: professional and mental health consumer/survivor researchers working together in a participatory action research project. *Psychiatr Rehabil J.* **25**: 379–87.
- Office of Science and Technology and the Wellcome Trust (2000) *Science and the Public: a review of science communication and public attitudes to science in Britain.* DTI and Wellcome Trust, London.
- Renfrew M and McCandlish R (1992) With women: new steps in research in midwifery. In: Roberts H (ed) *Women's Health Matters.* Routledge, London.
- Schwarcz SL (moderator) (1981) Non-scientist participation in the peer review process: Is it desirable? Is it implementable? Who are the non-scientists who should become involved? A panel discussion. *Ann NY Acad Sci.* **2**: 213–28.
- Sheppard B (2002) *Making a start: involving older people in the doctor's surgery.* Age Concern, London.
- Slevin ML, Stubbs L, Plant HJ *et al.* (1990) Attitudes to chemotherapy: comparing views of patients with cancer with those of doctors, nurses, and general public. *BMJ.* **300**: 1458–60.

- Tallon D, Chard J and Dieppe P (2000) Relation between agendas of the research community and the research consumer. *Lancet.* **355**: 2037–40.
- Thomas P (2000) The research needs of primary care: trials must be relevant to patients. *BMJ.* **321**: 2–3.
- Thornton H (1998) Alliance between medical profession and consumers already exists in breast cancer. *BMJ.* **316**: 148–9.
- Tighe RJ and Biersdorff KK (1993) Setting agendas for relevant research: a participatory approach. *Can J Rehab.* **7**: 127–32.
- Truman C and Raine P (2002) Experience and meaning of user involvement: some explorations from a community mental health project. *Health Soc Care Community.* **10**: 136–43.
- US Department of the Army (1998) *Congressionally Directed Medical Research Programs, Fiscal Year 1998. Status report.* US Army Medical Research and Material Command, 25, Fort Detrick, MD.
- Wensing M, Mainz J, Ferreira P *et al.* (1998) General practice care and patients' priorities in Europe: an international comparison. *Health Policy.* **45**: 175–86.
- Yearley S (1994) Understanding science from the perspective of the sociology of scientific knowledge: an overview. *Pub Underst Sci.* **3**: 245–58.

Chapter 3

Lay involvement: the who, what, where, when, why and how of involving lay people in research

Why lay involvement?

In 1992 the NHS Management Executive published a document called *Local Voices* indicating the importance of listening to local people in determining the nature of services to be purchased. These views were linked to the wider research evidence, the views and experiences of the locality. The Government's white paper of 1995 *The New NHS* asserts the aspiration to secure a strong public voice in health and healthcare decision making. The NHS Executive gave a further push in 1996 to involvement by promoting ideas about openness and accountability. Whilst these relate to services, the services should be based on the research. If there is to be more involvement in the service/delivery side there must be more involvement in the bedrock of these services: research.

Lay involvement can help:

- identify issues which are important to the wider community
- ensure focused research of practical relevance to the healthcare community
- enhance the opportunities for research funding
- provide new and intricate research challenges
- extend the researchers' repertoire
- vouch for research that measures processes and outcomes
- assure processes and outcomes are not solely seen from the clinician's perspective
- the recruitment of their associates and a wider community to the research programme
- access people who feel or are marginalised (e.g. some ethnic minorities, disabled, homeless, certain age groups, mentally infirm)

- access people in higher authority that the researchers could rarely reach themselves
- broadcast, disperse and disseminate the results of research
- provide impetus to help ensure that desired changes are implemented and audited.

Jane Daniels of the Clinical Trials Unit, University of Birmingham indicates (in a personal communication) that patient organisations can help 'access the higher echelons of the NHS/Department of Health that we could never reach directly and so can lobby on our behalf for the trials'. Citing the example of the Parkinson's Disease Society which is involved in some of the trials at the Birmingham Unit, Jane indicates that they also contribute to patient information sheets, promotion of the trials, understanding and conveying the issues and priorities of the target patient group, and sharing the attitudes of the clinical community more widely.

In the USA, the Congressionally Directed Medical Research Programs (CDMRP) became an important catalyst in the inclusion of lay involvement in peer review of scientific research from the mid-1990s. Whilst lay involvement included those who would be most affected by the proposed research, the findings of the CDMRP exercise suggest that:

- lay people felt that the scientists on their panel treated them with respect and acceptance, and appeared to value their contributions
- lay people believed the peer review process was fair, rigorous, and very positive
- lay people felt that they had made valuable contributions to the reviews
- scientists believed that a lay presence on peer review panels served as a reminder of the human dimensions of the disease
- scientists observed that the lay presence enhanced communication and that a mutual understanding between scientists and consumers was achieved.

Evidence such as this promoted the inclusion of lay people in research and they are now involved in major research funding bodies such as the National Institutes of Health and the National Cancer Institute. As a beacon of light, staff at the CDMRP have given assistance to various organisations such as the Canadian Breast Cancer Research Program, the National Cancer Institute, the National Institute of Mental Health, and the Network of Breast Cancer Research.

In Britain there is a growing bank of evidence on lay involvement in health, and emerging evidence of the ways in which lay involvement has made a difference to a project (*see* Table 3.1).

Table 3.1: Examples of the ways in which lay involvement has made a difference to a project

Title of topic	Making a difference
Cancer voices	The assumptions made about geographical areas for networking proved unrealistic so the consumers grounded the research in reality, related and networked within small geographical areas not necessarily coinciding with NHS regions
Patient and carer views of stroke services	The guideline included recommendations from patient/carer discussion groups
A randomised controlled trial to evaluate the benefit of a new information leaflet for parents of children hospitalised with benign febrile convulsions	Patients identified the need for and assisted in the production of a leaflet which reflected local practice
A large randomised long-term assessment of the relative cost-effectiveness of surgery for Parkinson's disease	The Parkinson's Disease Society emphasised the importance of research on patient-reported quality of life in addition to clinical measurements
Survey of views of people affected by motor neurone disease on the only drug treatment (then) available: riluzole	Made a questionnaire more user friendly
Evaluating the multiple sclerosis (MS) specialist nurse: a review and development of the role	Helped to ground the work in local reality. Helped to decide on two service standards as priority. Helped suggest ways in which the NHS nurse could develop a service to meet patient needs. Provided additional insights into the meaning of interview data and analysis
Torbay Healthy Housing Group: Watcombe Project	No evidence is yet available
Medication education	Changed the type of analysis, the instruments for measuring outcomes and assisted in the interpretation of the data
Befriending: more than just finding friends?	Helped select the correct words to use and ensured that all materials were accessible
Practice guidelines for primary healthcare teams to meet South Asian carers' needs	Involvement of bilingual interviews from the four main communities was vital in establishing links with the communities, recruiting carers who were caring in isolation, engendered trust in carers to voice their feelings and concerns about difficulties they encountered in caring for their relatives
What happens to people with severe aphasia?	There were major challenges with including people who cannot speak, read or write on advisory panel. This suggests skills facilitation, longer slower meetings with breaks, adapted minutes and agenda, and training for all panel members
Collaborative studies on health service and quality of life in people with learning disability	Information not yet in

Table 3.1: Continued

Title of topic	Making a difference
Joint replacement	Provided advice on who should have a joint replacement when the project was being piloted
Cognitive remediation: a randomised controlled trial	Experience with cognitive remediation was useful in helping design the patient satisfaction instrument
People's experiences of screening assessment by nurses in a community mental health team	They helped provide research data and critically appraised the literature on emerging models/theories
Disability equipment evaluations	The risk assessment of products prior to their evaluation in home trials resulted in the withdrawal of some products and determined what risk needed to be monitored in user trials
Cochrane skin group	Improved prioritisation of research and the readability of the review
Developing and evaluating best practice for user involvement in cancer services	In the same way as the rest of the team they contributed their ideas, experiences and expertise at project meetings where decisions are made about the research

Why do lay people choose to get involved in research?

To my mind it is just as important to understand why lay people want to be or are involved in research as it is to understand your reasons for wanting or having their involvement.

So why do lay people choose to get involved in research? Some reasons (not in rank order) include:

• altruism (for the greater good of society)
• natural curiosity
• to improve services
• to help identify problems and explore solutions
• to help make research more meaningful
• to support the local organisation
• to help prioritise research
• to offer opportunities for improving community ownership
• to aid public accountability, due process and transparency
• to provide insight from the outside
• to help shape good practice
• to help share good practice.

Can one or two lay people be representative of all laymen?

No. Just as it is often entirely unreasonable to think that any one doctor, nurse or pharmacist, represents all doctors, nurses and pharmacists, so it is entirely unreasonable to think that any one lay person, however well inclined and informed, can represent all lay people. A better approach is to look at it another way: do not think of it as lay representativeness but think of it as lay 'perspectives'. The more lay perspectives you want, the wider you will have to cast your net to secure lay people. Never dismiss a lay person's views just as their own – you cannot in fact prove it and you should not say it. To get around this think always of lay perspectives: never think of lay representativeness being completely representative even if some people do and others would like you to.

Can trained consumer advocates offer the views of 'typical' patients?

Maybe. These 'consumer groups' have skills, networks, experiences and histories of healthcare involvement, but unless they have recently sought the views of those you are interested in, in a systematic, transparent and robust manner, they will not be able to wholly reflect their views. They can however provide substantial insight into issues affecting say patients and clinical practice, and are often able to ask pertinent questions throughout their period of involvement in research. The example of the benefits of having the Parkinson's Disease Society involved in trials at the Clinical Trials Unit in Birmingham was indicated above.

Can health professionals act as lay people?

No. Not by definition, and not in practice. Despite their many good intentions and altruism, and despite a contention that they know a lot more about the healthcare system than 'outsider' lay people, health professionals are not the best source of a lay perspective. They use somewhat different languages, may have different priorities, have a lot of 'inside' healthcare experience, and may place different emphasis on the humanistic side of healthcare. Various authors, for instance, Allsop,

Frater, Grant-Pearce and colleagues, Kelson, Smith and Armstrong, Williamson,[1-6] show that mismatches can and do exist between the views and priorities of service providers (and researchers) and others in terms of the issues, needs, priorities, concerns and resolutions.

This does not mean other healthcare professionals cannot and should not be on the research team: if they are, then a decision has to be made, and made clear, about who they will represent, if anyone (e.g. their self, their profession, their organisation), and if it is their perspective or representativeness you are seeking in the research team enterprise.

Who should be involved?

Before venturing into the topic of who to involve as lay members in health research, let us step aside for a moment and look at the results of Davies'[7] work on lay involvement of eight statutory bodies regulating professionals in the health field. The objective of Davies' work was to find out what kind of people were appointed as lay members, their contributions and views of change. Davies also reports on 30–40 semi-structured interviews focusing on lay members' perceptions of regulatory tasks, their roles and accountability, their experiences, and their views on their distinctive contributions. What key messages can we take from this work (see Box 3.1)?

Let us look more closely at Davies' finding of lay members being from a narrow band of the population as this may have resonance for lay involvement in health research. Davies found that:

- few young people were involved (60% were over 55, no one was under 35)
- only 28% were in full-time work
- the split between males and females was in the ratio 60:40
- only 6.8% assigned themselves as being non-white
- most were high achievers, well known in their field
- three-quarters could be classified into the highest status occupational and social classes
- most had experienced public duties
- an NHS 'mafia' was evident – the majority had worked in the NHS
- three-quarters had no links to organisations representing health service users
- few had current active connections with service user groups that were campaigning for change and engaging with health issues locally.

Box 3.1: Lay involvement in health professional regulation

- Lay members are drawn from a narrow band of the population.
- Recruitment to posts has broadened in recent years. Formal processes are now in routine use and there is increasingly open advertisement of vacancies.
- Lay members, while they did not cite the growing consumer literature critical of current regulatory institutions, nonetheless echoed some of its concerns.
- Lay members were not convinced that the Government's modernisation agenda grappled with the key issues.
- Lay members strongly endorsed the need for and value of lay involvement.
- Lay members identified roles that they were able to play:
  - as a public guardian
  - challenging the narrow perspectives of professionals
  - asking apparently naive questions that teased out fundamental issues.
- Lay members resisted the notion that there were two camps of lay people and professionals, and argued it would be counter-productive to let this division occur.
- Absence of formal accountability was a major discussion point.
- Views differed on the merits and feasibility of broadening the recruitment of lay members.
- An alternative model of the roles, responsibility and relationships of a lay member was visible.
- The bodies with which lay members are involved are in an uneasy transition phase and in some ways change is at odds with public opinion.
- Areas for concern are:
  - selection and recruitment
  - terms and conditions
  - frameworks for training, mentoring and support
  - creation of lines of accountability and opportunities for group and individual performance review
  - new structures and processes to enhance lay involvement and dialogue with the public
  - closer working practices
  - commissioning of work that will foster joined-up thinking on lay participation.

Although there is, as yet, no similar study for lay involvement in health research, the information above gives some ideas on the data you can record in your research.

Before you attempt to answer the question of who to involve you must have identified the objectives of having lay involvement in your research. Prior to asking anyone to become involved in your research team you must be able to:

- explain the project in clear unambiguous terms
- indicate why you want lay involvement
- outline what is expected of lay members (e.g. time, input, resources, rewards, accountability, voting rights, parity, control)
- indicate what the benefits will be, where and when they are expected to arise.

These criteria do not just apply to work to be done before getting lay people involved, the same work should be done before you speak to possible research collaborators, potential funders, and the head of your host organisation. If you are a lay person and are invited to join a research project then start by asking the 'inviter' questions based on the above points.

In some cases I have seen job specifications drafted to help the researchers frame their ideas about the type of person and expectations of the lay member(s). In other cases, the researcher has gone to certain groups of people and asked them their views on certain issues – giving the researcher vignettes upon which to help establish a framework to rebuild an account of the research team's roles and responsibilities.

Other sources of input to the research plan can be garnered by inviting, or at least listening to, perspectives from:

- self-help groups
- voluntary organisations
- pressure groups
- advocacy groups.

Table 3.2 provides a variety of examples of who was involved in certain projects.

Table 3.2: Examples of who was involved

Title of topic	Examples of who was involved
Cancer voices	Cancer service users and carers, mostly from cancer self-help and support groups
Patient and carer views of stroke services	Representatives from the College of Health Stroke Association; members of local stroke groups participated in the discussion groups
A randomised controlled trial to evaluate the benefit of a new information leaflet for parents of children hospitalised with benign febrile convulsions	A local parent information group within the trust
A large randomised long-term assessment of the relative cost-effectiveness of surgery for Parkinson's disease	Parkinson's Disease Society (PDS) representatives
Survey of views of people affected by motor neurone disease on the only drug treatment (then) available: riluzole	Members of the Motor Neurone Disease Association, people with the disease, carers and past carers
Evaluating the multiple sclerosis (MS) specialist nurse: a review and development of the role	People with MS, carers, members of local and national MS voluntary groups
Torbay Healthy Housing Group: Watcombe Project	Residents on a council estate
Medication education	Service user from the trust was involved in the research team. Service users from the trust asked for the medication education service
Befriending: more than just finding friends?	A group of young people helping to develop the leaflets and design the questionnaire
Practice guidelines for primary healthcare teams to meet South Asian carers' needs	Male and female bilingual interviewers were recruited and trained from the four main communities
What happens to people with severe aphasia?	People with severe aphasia, their families, speech language therapists, voluntary sector workers, organisations of disabled people and their self-help groups
Collaborative studies on health service and quality of life in people with learning disability	A user–carer agency forum has been convened, drawn from service users, parents, carers, advocates, representatives from the private and voluntary sector providers, social and religious organisations
Joint replacement	Mainly recruited from the hospital clinics and some from the general practice sector
Cognitive remediation: a randomised controlled trial	Consumers of previous studies of cognitive remediation
People's experiences of screening assessment by nurses in a community mental health team	Service users with recent experiences of assessment
Disability equipment evaluations	Members of voluntary groups (e.g. stroke club), social service clients, health service outpatients and individuals in residential homes
Cochrane skin group	Twenty-two members of the National Eczema Society and the UK Cochrane Centre
Developing and evaluating best practice for user involvement in cancer services	Two representatives from voluntary organisations (Cancerlink and Bristol Cancer Help Centre) and service user representatives

How many lay people should I involve? (One is a lonely number)

There are many benefits from involving more than one lay person in a particular research project. For example, suppose you have two lay people involved in your research team then at best they can:

- offer each other mutual support
- reduce isolation
- share lay ideas
- clarify roles and responsibilities of themselves and others in the team
- confirm interpretation of issues and events
- corroborate decisions and understanding
- increase self-confidence
- reduce the burden on you
- improve team confidence and team spirit
- enhance self-esteem
- still provide lay input if one lay person drops out
- provide new and exciting public relations opportunities
- open up new possibilities of linking into other networks.

I simply suggest that you get involved with outside groups even if you are not doing any research just now. In this way you will build up fruitful relationships and generate wonderfully rich insights into healthcare issues, or issues affecting healthcare, well before the genesis of any research exercise.

What type of involvement do I want?

The type of involvement could and does vary. For example, Clayton and colleagues[8] suggested four types of involvement:

- Passive: where lay people basically welcome the research proposals and support them but are not involved in the decision making
- Consultative: where lay people are consulted by professionals about their opinions and/or knowledge
- Active: where lay people play the role of active partners in the project and assume some responsibility
- Ownership: where lay people are both willing and able to have or take control of the project.

Much of the current lay involvement strategies involve passive, consultative or active involvement.

When should lay members be involved?

Some of the best examples of lay involvement are where lay involvement has started before a research project is designed. The lay involvement can of course still be successful even if it comes in at other stages of the research.

Reading down the first column of Table 3.3 gives you a flavour of the different stages where lay involvement can become a part of the research. In Table 3.3 I have added four columns for the 'types' of involvement e.g. passive, consultative. By setting the table out in this way it suggests to me that you can use it to identify what type of involvement you would prefer and at what stages of the research. In fact Tables 3.3 and 3.4 can also be used to generate discussions in the research team of the type and stage of involvement, and as a mapping exercise to trace and record what type of involvement took place at certain stages during the life of the project.

Table 3.3: Some stages and types of lay involvement

	Type of involvement			
Stage of involvement	*Passive*	*Consultative*	*Active*	*Ownership*
1 Identifying topics				
2 Prioritising				
3 Submitting application forms (e.g. to ethics committees, funding bodies, heads of research host organisation)				
4 Recruiting and additional fundraising				
5 Planning				
6 Designing				
7 Undertaking				
8 Managing				
9 Disseminating				
10 Follow-up work, including evaluation of impact				

Table 3.4: **Examples of stages of involvement**

Title of topic	Examples of stages of involvement
Cancer voices	• Prioritising topic area • Planning the research
Patient and carer views of stroke services	• Planning the research • Managing the research • Designing the research instruments • Analysing the research • Writing publications • Disseminating the research
A randomised controlled trial to evaluate the benefit of a new information leaflet for parents of children hospitalised with benign febrile convulsions	• Prioritising topic areas
A large randomised long-term assessment of the relative cost-effectiveness of surgery for Parkinson's disease	• Funding, prioritising topic areas • Disseminating the research • Implementing action
Survey of views of people affected by motor neurone disease on the only drug treatment (then) available: riluzole	• Prioritising research area • Designing the research instruments
Evaluating the multiple sclerosis (MS) specialist nurse: a review and development of the role	• Prioritising topic areas • Designing research instruments • Analysing the research • Identifying local organisations and key individuals to consult
Torbay Healthy Housing Group: Watcombe Project	• Planning the research • Randomisation of houses to be upgraded • Managing the research
Medication education	• Prioritising topic areas • Planning the research • Managing the research • Designing the research instruments • Undertaking the research • Analysing the research • Writing publications • Disseminating the research • Implementing action
Befriending: more than just finding friends?	• Designing the research instruments • Disseminating the research
Practice guidelines for primary healthcare teams to meet South Asian Carers' needs	• Designing the research instruments • Undertaking the research • Preliminary analysis of the research • Undertaking focus groups and in-depth interviews • Disseminating the research
What happens to people with severe aphasia?	• Prioritising topic areas • Planning the research • Managing the research • Designing the research instruments • Analysing the research
Collaborative studies on health service and quality of life in people with learning disability	• Prioritising topic areas • Managing the research • Designing the research instruments • Disseminating the research • Implementing action

Table 3.4: Continued

Title of topic	Examples of stages of involvement
Joint replacement	• Planning the research
Cognitive remediation: a randomised controlled trial	• Designing the research instruments
	• Undertaking the research
People's experiences of screening assessment by nurses in a community mental health team	• Analysing the research
	• Writing publications
Disability equipment evaluations	• Prioritising topic areas
	• Planning the research
	• Designing the research instruments
Cochrane skin group	• Prioritising topic areas
	• Planning the research
	• Managing the research
	• Undertaking the research
	• Analysing the research
	• Writing publications
Developing and evaluating best practice for user involvement in cancer services	• Planning the research
	• Designing the research instruments
	• Undertaking the research
	• Writing publications
	• Disseminating the research

How can lay people be identified?

First of all, think about what type of person you want to involve. You do not need to know the person specifically but you do need to know if they are patients, ex-patients, carers, family relatives of patients or carers, a young person, people with special needs, long-term users of services, members of community groups, consumer advocates, and other lay people.

In terms of identifying lay people outside your organisation, various additional sources of advice exist and should be considered:

• local voluntary services
• local organisations e.g. for the elderly, mentally ill, single mothers, homeless, ethnic and minority groups
• patient forums (developed from local community health councils)
• local authorities
• the Health Information Service
• the World Wide Web (e.g. especially the consumer in research website)
• NHS organisations – NHS research and development regional offices, GPs' surgeries
• College of Health Self Help Group Directory
• local libraries
• race equality councils

- colleagues who have used lay people before
- patient and local community networks
- funding organisations who may have lists of contacts and ideas on how to approach lay people
- outside healthcare organisations (e.g. public, private, charitable) where lay perspectives have been used
- advertising on local notice-boards
- producing research information on posters and in exhibitions
- holding formal and informal 'meet the researchers' gatherings
- advertising through other local media and newsletters.

According to Muhib and colleagues from Boston,[9] constructing scientifically sound samples of hard-to-reach populations is a challenge for many projects. Traditional sample survey methods, such as random sampling from telephone or mailing lists, can yield low numbers of eligible respondents while non-probability sampling introduces unknown biases. One method that can be used to help overcome this is a venue-based application of time-space sampling (TSS). Simply put, the method entails identifying days and times when the target population gathers at specific venues, constructing a sampling frame, randomly selecting and visiting venues, and systematically intercepting and collecting information from consenting members of the target population. Carefully done this will allow you to construct a sample with known properties, make statistical inference to the larger population of venue visitors, and theorise about the introduction of biases that may limit generalisation of results.

Smith and colleagues from the Wake Forest University School of Medicine explored the value of community collaboration in a qualitative study of diabetes.[10] Using state-wide focus groups, the researchers benefited by gaining entry to communities, and the community organisations benefited by gaining a better understanding of the diabetic population to assist in planning programmes. Smith and colleagues argue that the identification and involvement of trusted, accessible members of rural communities gives research local legitimacy, ensures adequate participation and effective data collection, and permits entry into remote communities.[10]

Payment to lay members

Why bother paying lay members?

Lay members will be expected to attend meetings, spend time analysing material, talking through documents, travelling, covering dependants' costs and so on. Paying lay members brings into play the possibility of equity amongst the research team. For example, few if any of the other members of the research team will be providing their time, expertise and energies for nothing, so why should lay members not be paid? Payment could also improve the chances of recruiting and retaining good quality lay members to the research team. Payment may be used to help spell out what is expected of the lay members. And finally, payment is a small token way of putting some value on the lay contributions.

What should you consider paying for?

I think it best to outline a menu of things I have seen paid for:

- travel
- accommodation
- subsistence
- telephone/fax/Internet expenses
- stationery and equipment
- relevant training and mentoring
- conference/workshop costs
- childcare/costs of using a carer (e.g. to facilitate the lay member attending the meetings etc.)
- time off work/college/school.

Best practice suggests that in the plan for the research budget you make it clear what is going to be paid, to whom, when and at what rate.

You should certainly be very careful if you are planning to pay by result – the reasons being that few others in the team are paid that way; the results are always hard to identify; finding a causal relationship between individual effort and any particular result is prone to many flaws, analysis paralysis, and needless time-consuming arguments.

How much should I pay?

There is no fixed universal rate of payment so maybe lessons can be learnt from others that are paying. Here are some examples (in alphabetical order).

- Department of Health Strategic Review of NHS R&D in Mental Health paid £150 to members of the specially convened user panel for their attendance plus expenses.
- Devon Social Services offer £50 for attending a full-day meeting, half that rate for half-day meetings.

- Gedling Primary Care Trust pays £95 to lay members participating in meetings.
- Joseph Rowntree Foundation offers £75 per meeting, if unwaged, plus additional amounts for preparation time, and support workers.
- NHS HTA pays £122 a day for attending panel meetings, including induction/training days. HTA also pays travel, subsistence and carer costs.
- National Lotteries Charities Board pays user assessors of social and medical research a fee of £125 plus expenses, the same as other assessors.
- NICE suggests that it will be paying £150 per day to members of its newly formed 'Citizens Council'.
- Wiltshire and Swindon Users' Network set up a limited company to cover, amongst other things, the payment of users' costs.

Are there any other issues to consider in paying lay members?

Yes.

- Give the lay members the choice of receiving payment in cash/bank credit or paying the same amount of money to say a charity of their choice.
- Take into account the lay members' financial situation (tax and state benefits) e.g. especially if they are retired, registered unemployed, registered disabled or self-employed.
- Payments must be prompt. In some of the best cases, payments were made in advance and fine calculations were carried out at the end of the year to cover any underpayment.
- Think about making payment rules and schedules transparent: but if you do this for lay members you must also do this for all the other members of the research team. Apart from being financially prudent it also offers good signals of financial stewardship.

Make sure you have advanced agreement with the sponsor of the research and the ethics committee before you agree to any payment system.

Confidentiality

Some of those who resist lay involvement in research cite concern about confidentiality. Two lines of argument are:

- the more people involved in research the greater the likelihood of breaches in confidentiality

- those subject to the research, e.g. patients in the clinical trial, will be less confident when more people are involved in the research team.

There is no robust evidence to support any of these concerns, but since they are concerns, they need attention. Probably the best solution is to make all those involved in the research aware of the Data Protection Act, the Declaration of Helsinki and the Caldicott principles on data handling.[11] It would also be good practice for the leaders of the research to write up a code of practice on confidentiality, and to get every individual in the research team to sign that agreement. It is important that lay members understand the confidentiality issues, how they will be handled in the research programme, and what is expected of them. Some people do not appreciate or understand where the confidential information can end up, so advanced thinking and planning around issues of confidentiality is essential.

Indeed lay members may be amongst some of the strongest and loudest voices in the research team, motivated to help ensure confidentiality is secured and seen to be secured in the project.

Complexity

Can lay members understand and make good use of what can become complex data and management issues in a research project? To be frank it really depends on the individuals you bring into the research team, their induction programme, and how they are subsequently handled. No two lay members will be exactly alike. Lay members are not homogenous people, readily brought off a shelf just when you need them. They need to be recruited carefully, trained professionally, and valued like any other member of the research team. Lay members can bring into the research team a rich diversity of knowledge, analytical reasoning, questioning and inquisition beyond that which clinical researchers can or do themselves provide in the research.

Medico-legal issues of lay involvement in research

Given the inexorable rise in litigation in healthcare and the growing use of lay members in research, one would have thought that there would be a bank of evidence available surrounding the medico-legal issues of lay involvement in research. After contacting various medico-legal experts, the Medical Defence Union, the Department of Health, and funding bodies, the only advice that can be offered is that the lay members are subject to the same medico-legal issues as any other normal member of the research team would be.

If, and it is only if, there are any details in a particular research contract with the lay member to suggest otherwise, then that must be made transparent, explained, and confirmed by legal experts. Best practice suggests to me that any such caveats must also be cleared with the funders of the research, the host institution, the relevant ethics committees, and of course be told to the patients in the research, and other research members.

The best and safest prospect is to have parity in the research team so all are subject to the same rules and regulations covering the medico-legal issues. It is important that lay members understand the medico-legal issues and what is expected of them as a member of the research team.

References

1 Allsop J (1996) The NHS and its users. In: J Campling (ed) *Health Policy and the NHS Towards 2000*. Longman, London.

2 Frater A (1992) Health outcomes: a challenge to the status quo. *Qual in Healthcare*. **1**: 87–8.

3 Grant-Pearce C, Miles I and Hill PI (1998) *Mismatches in priorities for health research between professionals and consumers*. Policy Research in Engineering, Science and Technology paper. University of Manchester, Manchester.

4 Kelson M (1997) *User Involvement. A Guide to Developing Effective User Involvement Strategies in the NHS*. College of Health, London.

5 Smith C and Armstrong D (1989) Comparison of criteria derived by government and patients for evaluating general practitioner services. *BMJ*. **299**: 494–6.

6 Williamson C (1992) *Whose standards: consumer and professional standards in healthcare*. Open University Press, Buckingham.

7 Davies CM (2001) *Lay Involvement in Professional Regulation*. Report from the School of Health and Social Welfare, Open University, Milton Keynes.

8 Clayton A, Oakley P and Pratt B (1997) *Empowering People: A guide to participation*. INTRAC, Oxford.

9 Muhib FB, Lin LS, Stueve A *et al.* (2001) *A venue based method for sampling hard-to-reach populations*. Public Health Report 116, Suppl. 1: 216–22.

10 Smith SL, Blake K, Olson CR and Tessaro I (2002) Community entry in conducting rural focus groups: process, legitimacy and lessons learned. *J Rural Health.* **18**: 118–23.

11 Caldicott Committee (1997) *Report on the Review of Patient Identifiable Information.* Department of Health, London.

Further reading

- Arnstein SR (1969) A ladder of citizen participation. *Journal of American Institute of Planners.* **35**(4): 216–61.
- Barnes M and Warren L (eds) (1999) *Paths to Empowerment.* The Policy Press, Bristol.
- Baxter L, Thorne L and Mitchell A (2001) *Small Voices: big noises: lay involvement in health research: lessons from other fields.* Folk.us Programme, University of Exeter, Exeter.
- Buckland S and Entwistle V (2000) *Suggested Guidance for Grant Applicants About Involving Consumers in Research.* Consumers in NHS Research, Eastleigh, Hampshire.
- Chalmers I (1995) What do I want from health research and researchers when I am a patient? *BMJ.* **310**: 1315–18.
- Coats AJ (2000) Consumer involvement in cardiovascular research: ways to combat bias and secrecy. *Int J Cardiol.* **75**: 1–3.
- Congressionally Directed Medical Research Programs (2002) *How Can Other Organizations Set Up a Program to Involve Consumers?* CDMRP, Maryland, USA.
- Consumers in NHS Research (2002) *A Guide to Paying Consumers Actively Involved in Research.* Consumers in NHS Research Support Unit, Eastleigh, Hampshire.
- Department of Health (2002) *Consumer Involvement: consumers in NHS research.* Department of Health, London.
- Department of Health (1999) *Patient and Public Involvement in the New NHS.* Department of Health, London.
- Dwyer J (1989) The politics of participation. *Comm Health Studies.* **13**: 59–65.
- Earl-Slater A (2002) *The Handbook of Clinical Trials and Other Research.* Radcliffe Medical Press, Oxford.
- Entwistle V, Renfrew M, Yearly S *et al.* (1998) Lay perspectives: advantages for health research. *BMJ.* **316**: 463–6.
- Entwistle VA, Sheldon TA, Sowden AJ *et al.* (1996) Supporting consumer involvement in decision making: what constitutes quality in consumer health information? *Int J Qual Health Care.* **8**: 425–37.
- Evans C and Carmichael A (2002) *Users Best Value: a guide to user involvement good practice in best value reviews.* York Publishing Services, York.

- Flanagan J (1999) Public participation in the design of educational programmes for cancer nurses: a case report. *Eur J Cancer Care.* **8**: 107–12.
- Fleming B and Golding L (1997) *Involving Users* vol. 1. Soundings Research, Birmingham.
- Folk.us (2002) *Understanding Users as Trainers: facilitators as trainers' voices.* Folk.us Programme, University of Exeter, Exeter.
- Folk.us (2002) *Understanding Users as Trainers: users' voices.* Folk.us Programme, University of Exeter, Exeter.
- Goodare H and Smith R (1995) The rights of patients in research. *BMJ.* **310**: 1277–8.
- Groome PA, Hutchinson TA and Tousignant P (1994) Content of a decision analysis for treatment choice in end stage renal disease: who should be consulted? *Br J Gen Pract.* **14**: 91–7.
- Hanley B, on behalf of the Standing Group on Consumers in NHS Research (1999) *Involvement Works: the second report of the Standing Group on Consumers in NHS Research.* Department of Health, London.
- Hanley B (1999) Research and development in the NHS: how can you make a difference? *Health Expect.* **2**: 72.
- Harrison A and New B (2001) The finance of research and development in healthcare. In: J Appleby and A Harrison (eds) *Health Care UK 2001.* King's Fund, London.
- Heller T, Pederson EL and Miller AB (1996) Guidelines from the consumer: improving consumer involvement in research and training for persons with mental retardation. *Ment Retard.* **34**: 141–8.
- Help for Health Trust (undated) *Training for Professionals, lay representatives and consumers.* The Help for Health Trust, Winchester, Hampshire.
- House of Lords Select Committee on Science and Technology (1995) *Medical Research and the NHS Reforms.* HL Paper 12, Session 1994–5, 3rd report. HMSO, London.
- Irwin A (1995) *Citizen Science: a study of people, expertise and sustainable development.* Routledge, London.
- Jakubowska D and Crossley P (1999) Developing skills in consulting with the public. *BMJ.* **319**: 2–3.
- Kelson M (1998) *Promoting Consumer Involvement in Clinical Audit: practical guidelines on achieving effective involvement.* College of Health, London.
- De Koning K and Martin M (eds) (1996) *Participatory Research in Health.* Zed Books, London.
- Liberati A (1997) Consumer participation in research and health care: making it a reality. *BMJ.* **315**: 499.
- Local Management Government Board (1994) *Community Participation in Local Agenda 21.* Local Government Management Board (Local agenda 21 round table guidance), Luton.
- Matrice D and Brown V (eds) (1990) *Widening the Research Focus: consumer roles in public health research.* Consumers' Health Forum of Australia, Canberra.

- McNeill PM, Berglund CA and Webster IW (1994) How much influence do various members have within research ethics committees? *Camb Q Healthc Ethics*. Special Section: Research Ethics. **3**: 522–32.
- Morris J (1996) *Encouraging User Involvement in Commissioning: a resource for commissioners*. NHS Executive/Department of Health, Leeds.
- National Institute for Clinical Excellence (NICE) (2002) *A Short Introduction to the Citizens Council*. NICE, London.
- Newell C (1992) Consumer participation in the bioethics of disability. *Health Forum*. **22**: 11–13.
- North West Regional R&D Office (2002) *How Can We Involve Users in Research?* (a report of three conferences held in 2000). R&D Directorate, North West Regional R&D Office, Warrington.
- North West Regional R&D Office (2002) *Making it Happen: action planning for user involvement in R&D* (a report of an action research workshop held in April 2001). R&D Directorate, North West Regional R&D Office, Warrington.
- North West Regional R&D Office (2002) *Training for Service User Involvement in NHS Research and Development* (summary of training focus group workshops to develop a training programme for users). R&D Directorate, North West Regional R&D Office, Warrington.
- North West Regional R&D Office (2002) *User Involvement in NHS Provider Organisations* (a report of trusts in receipt of support funding). R&D Directorate, North West Regional R&D Office, Warrington.
- Nowak R (1995) AIDS researchers, activists, fight crisis in clinical trials. *Science*. **269**: 1666–7.
- Ochocka J, Janzen R and Nelson G (2002) Sharing power and knowledge: professional and mental health consumer/survivor researchers working together in a participatory action research project. *Psychiatr Rehabil J*. **25**: 379–87.
- Oliver SR (1995) How can health service users contribute to the NHS research and development programme? *BMJ*. **310**: 1318–20.
- Ong BN (1996) The lay perspective in health technology assessment. *Int J Technol Assess Health Care*. **12**: 511–17.
- Pfeffer N (1994) Creating dialogues: community health councils. In: Dunning M and Needham G (eds) *But Will It Work, Doctor?* Report of a conference about involving users of health services in outcomes research. The Consumer Health Information Consortium, Winchester.
- Rockwell GR (1993) The role and function of the public member. *Federation Bulletin*. Spring: 42–4.
- Royle J, Steel R, Hanley B *et al.* (undated) *Getting Involved in Research: a guide for consumers*. Consumers in NHS Research Support Unit, Eastleigh, Hampshire.
- Russell H and Szoke H (1990) *Review of Consumer Participation in the National Health and Medical Research Council*. Consumers' Health Forum of Australia, Canberra.

- Sheppard B (2002) *Making a Start: involving older people in the doctor's surgery.* Age Concern, London.
- Simeonsson RJ, Edmondson R, Smith T *et al.* (1995) Family involvement in multidisciplinary team evaluation: professional and parent perspectives. *Child Care Health Dev.* **21**: 199–214 (comment 214–15).
- Standing Group on Consumers in NHS Research (1999) *Strategic Alliances Workshop 27 January 1999: workshop report.* Help for Health Trust, Winchester.
- Telford R (2002) *Successful Consumer Involvement in Research: an evaluation using consensus-generated criteria.* School of Health and Related Research, Sheffield.
- Thorne L, Putsell R and Baxter L (2001) *Knowing How – a guide to getting involved in research.* Folk.us, Exeter University CNHSR, Exeter.
- Thornton H (1998) Alliance between medical profession and consumers already exists in breast cancer. *BMJ.* **316**: 148–9.
- Thornton H (1995) *The Patients' Role in Research.* In: Health Committee, Third Report vol. II. HMSO, London.
- Wadsworth Y (1990) The consumer contribution to public health research and its funding administration. In: Matrice D and Brown V (eds) *Widening the Research Focus: consumer roles in public health research.* Consumers' Health Forum of Australia, Canberra.
- Williamson C (2001) What does involving consumers in research mean? *Q J Med.* **94**: 661–4.

Chapter 4

Lay involvement strategies

There are many ways to have lay involvement in research and what follows is a brief outline of some of the strategies that have been used in the UK and overseas.

Lay involvement strategies

Various authors have provided alternative guidance on lay involvement frameworks.[1-3] Dixon and colleagues not only provide classification of the types and areas of involvement, but suggest a rating scale to measure the extent of the involvement.[1] Entwistle and colleagues provide a framework on the stages of research, possible involvement contributions, and ways of identifying and involving people in the research.[2] Hanley and colleagues indicate various reasons for research involvement, types, stages and processes of possible involvement.[3]

Ideally you need to choose the strategy which is considered the best conceivable one to help achieve the objectives of lay involvement in the research exercise. Best practice suggests that the basis of the decision should be made:

- after you have spoken to consumer advocacy groups (either consumer advocates in general or those with particular disease/service area experience you are researching in)
- after you have spoken to colleagues in your organisation about their views and experiences
- after you have spoken to other researchers in the field
- after you have spoken to the potential funders of the research about their rules, regulations, requirements, and of course
- after you have read any reviews of the accumulating evidence of lay involvement in research projects.

Do not choose a strategy just because it is 'what we did last year, what my colleague is doing', or the 'fashionable thing to do'. Remember you only have a certain amount of goodwill and trust in your own life, and consumers only have a certain amount of goodwill, patience and trust that they can offer. Do not rush into choosing a lay involvement strategy, as the wrong strategy will do you, your colleagues, your organisation, your sponsors, lay members and most importantly your research subjects a serious disservice.

Whilst some of the elements of lay involvement strategies are outlined in Box 4.1, categorised individually, they are not mutually exclusive: you can have a mixture of them. You can have them running at different times of your research programme. There is certainly no reason why you yourself should be responsible for running a portfolio of strategies chosen. In some cases I have seen lay involvement programmes where all the main strategies below were pre-planned along a timescale and successfully accomplished, some being run by people other than the lead researcher.

Box 4.1: Elements and types of lay involvement strategies

- Regular community meetings
- Community liaison networks
- Mentorships
- As resource people
- As members of advisory panels
- As non-voting members of research projects
- As voting members of research projects
- As teaching beneficiaries – e.g. to provide students direct opportunities to hear them as a teacher/educator/informer
- Invitations to seminars, presentations and workshops

Factors helping or hindering lay involvement

Box 4.2 provides an outline of some factors that may help or indeed hinder lay involvement in research. It is important to think of these whilst you are designing and developing a lay involvement strategy. This will help you to ensure that lay involvement is not tokenism, and to dilute any intimidation lay members may feel in coming into the research team.

Box 4.2: Factors helping or hindering lay involvement

Attitudes

Attitudes of professionals towards lay involvement in research can help or hinder lay involvement. Where the funders have a more benevolent and positive attitude towards lay involvement this acts as a facilitator. If the research team includes professionals who are not welcoming, then it will benefit no one if their attitude does not change, and change quickly. The lead researcher and the chairman, if not the same person, must have a positive, constructive, innovative and welcoming attitude to lay involvement for it to be a success.

Management

Some research team managers are excellent, but some are not. Linked to attitudes, it is clear which type of manager will facilitate and which will only serve to frustrate lay involvement in the research.

Diversity

The diversity and complexity within and between people is often overlooked. There are systematic techniques that can be used to ensure lay involvement captures much of that diversity and complexity.

Knowledge

Lay people have their own knowledge base just as the rest of the research team do. Professionals may lack local knowledge and compassion and lay people may lack knowledge of the research. Both knowledge bases can be garnered and managed in a constructive mutually beneficial way.

Power

Power relationships abound. Many professionals and researchers believe they are pioneering and their work should be fully funded without question. Potential and actual funders have limited funds and must invest wisely. Patients are the subjects of research and may feel overpowered by the halo of being in a research project and apprehensive about yet more involvement in the research through lay people. Lay people may feel least powerful in the team unless given equal voting rights, equal access to documents, and equal time to ask questions.

Resources
Lack of time, funds, materials, knowledge, information, experience, and poor training opportunities are often cited as barriers to lay involvement. Some projects have successfully recruited and retained lay involvement by paying lay people on the same basis they pay others in the research team.

Trust
Trust must be earned, visible and documented. Professionals should trust lay involvement in their research and lay people should trust that they will be told the truth at all times.

Values
Professional groups must become less protective of 'their territory' because it is basically not theirs. Rather than see lay involvement as yet another trespass, intrusion or invasion, it should be seen as opportunities to build better, more productive, more useful research. Honesty and openness facilitate lay involvement.

Successful lay involvement in research programmes

Lay involvement in research is on the increase but there is, as yet, no robust evidence that identifies the characteristics of any successful lay involvement programme. By 'successful' I mean that the programme is successful, not simply or exclusively that the lay member is successful in whatever they have done in the particular research programme.

Define why you need lay involvement

Are you looking for lay involvement to enhance the research services that you provide, to strengthen your community involvement, to enrich your exposure to certain communities? Is there a genuine reason to use lay involvement? State it crisply and clearly. Every lay involvement programme must begin with an understanding of why you and your organisation want or need lay involvement support. Ensure that you have the support of your superiors before embarking on a lay involvement recruitment campaign. It is essential to establish desired outcomes for lay involvement. Establishing these outcome objectives early in the enterprise will help to guide the types of lay members that you recruit, and the way that you manage them once they have come on board.

Design valuable lay involvement opportunities

By designing valuable lay involvement assignments you provide lay involvement with clear challenges and motivation for continued success. You also provide a structure on which others in the research team know and can gauge their involvement. Set out the responsibilities of each job. Build in adequate training and support programmes to facilitate lay involvement learning and development, and ensure that lay members are aware of the goals and outcome objectives of their involvement.

Recruit carefully

When you have designed your lay involvement opportunities, target the appropriate audiences to recruit those who are interested in the research project. As foundation work, understand the characteristics of your existing team, and recruit lay involvement to mirror this team. Be honest to everyone about the workload and time commitment involved in the project. Above all, ask for help but never plead – you want lay members who want to be there.

Screen, interview and place cautiously

Screening and interviewing potential lay members can boost their commitment to the research project. How? It shows potential lay members and the rest of the research team that you take both the project and their time seriously. Screening also gives you an opportunity to match qualifications and skills with your needs. An interview is probably the best time to define availability and schedule activities that fit both the research project and lay members' involvement.

Bring lay members on board with training

Comprehensive orientation and lay involvement induction and training programmes give lay members a feeling of belonging and status. It shows that you value them enough to make an investment in them and, again, helps to reinforce their commitment to the cause. Orientation also helps set the tone of the work area and allows lay members to adapt more easily to the research team's surroundings.

As part of the lay involvement training sessions, you should provide a general orientation to the research, including a discussion of its mission and philosophy. Outline the research framework and any codes of conduct that are enforceable. Offer project-specific training that is necessary to develop skills and confidence.

The three Rs: recognise, respect, reward

You must have thought about recognition programmes before you begin to secure and nurture lay involvement. Recognition shows that you and your research team value lay involvement. Recognition programmes offer another motivation for continuing commitment from lay members in the research. Recognition can be formal or informal: best practice suggests it should be a combination of these. Remember that public relations exercises and annual reports of research progress can be improved, and in some cases vastly improved, by adding in the lay members' contributions.

Respect must be two-way: from you to the lay members and from the lay members to the rest of the team involved in the research. If there is any concern about lack of respect, find out who holds that concern, what it is, why it is held, and what if anything can be done about it. Do not take respect for granted: it must be built up, nurtured, justified, and visible.

Rewards must be appropriate to the input that the lay members have provided. However, when looking at the three Rs do not forget the rest of the research team, otherwise you will be acting inequitably: recognise, respect and reward each individual and the team as a team.

Effective and efficient follow-up

Another element of a successful lay involvement programme is continual follow-up and careful evaluation. Effective and efficient follow-up provides feedback to everyone involved in the research about decisions and progress being made. It offers opportunities for reflection and refinement, planning and administration. Properly set out, well recorded, and carefully assessed lay involvement should not be difficult to assess.

Programme leadership

The lay involvement programme needs a good leader and a competent team. Experience, conviction, honesty, integrity and energy are paramount.

Vision, strategy, objectives and planning

Tight deadlines are needed for a limited number of clear objectives, explicit milestones, constant review and monitoring. These should help generate unwavering interest in keeping the programme on track. A robust and clear research business plan is required.

Staff

High calibre appointments are needed with careful attention to skill mix, explicit rewards and penalties, technical support and clear communications. The research programme leader must be an ambassador and all other members of the research team must act as diplomats.

Training

Continuous training in a structured manner is required, to develop an affinity with the ideas, strengths and weaknesses of lay involvement and management. Training should include in-house training (e.g. mentorship) and external training to help build and maintain competencies, enthusiasm, efficiency and effectiveness.

Records

Systematic, readable, catalogued and audited records should always be kept. Details of meetings and documents imported from outside the research team should be dealt with in a similar manner.

Communication

All members of the research programme should be clear as to the goals of the programme and their own value within it. It must be clear who has what authority to deal with communications with people outside the programme. It must be clear what action has to take place if a communication channel breaks down. Consistency in good communication is essential.

Relationship building

The programme leader must constantly build and reinforce relationships with people outside the research programme. The programme team must be able to relate to all others in the team. New ways of communication with outsiders must always be assessed in terms of the programme's objectives.

Every research programme with lay involvement should have **SMART** objectives:

- **S**pecific
- **M**easurable
- **A**ttainable but challenging
- **R**elevant
- **T**ime-orientated.

Box 4.3 provides an outline of possible attributes of a successful lay involvement research programme. I say 'possible attributes' because no one has actually provided a robust analysis of the growing case material to find out the actual ingredients of successful lay involvement in research programmes. Nevertheless, I have found these attributes in other research programmes and I have every confidence that some if not all of these attributes, and more, will be seen to be distinguishing features of successful research programmes involving lay members.

These are keys to successful lay involvement in research, not guarantees.

Widely adapted from the work of Walshe and colleagues, Box 4.4 provides an agenda for action for lay involvement in research in the form of a series of questions.[4] Maybe as an exercise you can attempt to answer these questions for your own research and see what transpires. In fact if you do this, why not share your results with a wider audience by publishing them?

Box 4.3: Key ingredients of successful lay involvement in research programmes

- Define why you need lay involvement
- Design valuable lay involvement opportunities
- Recruit carefully
- Screen, interview and place cautiously
- Bring lay members on board with training
- The three Rs: recognise, respect, reward
- Effective and efficient follow-up
- Programme leadership
- Vision, strategy, objectives and planning
- Staff
- Training
- Records
- Communication
- Relationship building

Box 4.4: An agenda for action for lay involvement in research

- Is the host organisation's board really involved in and genuinely committed to lay involvement?
- Is there an executive director on the board who takes full responsibility for improving lay involvement?
- Does the organisation have a formal strategy for lay involvement?
- Is there a co-ordinating group responsible for leading on lay involvement?
- Is there a senior individual working with the lead executive director to implement a strategy on lay involvement?
- Has the organisation reviewed its structure in the light of its strategy for improving lay involvement?
- Does the organisation have adequate access to information resources?
- How does the organisation disseminate and follow up information on lay involvement?
- Is appropriate training relating to lay involvement being provided?
- Are health authorities incorporating evidence on lay involvement into their key roles in assessing healthcare needs, and commissioning services to meet those needs?

- Are trusts gathering and incorporating evidence of lay involvement effectiveness into their key roles in healthcare?
- Is the progress of efforts to improve lay involvement and to foster evidence-based lay involvement regularly monitored and reviewed?
- Are efforts to improve lay involvement having a measurable effect?

References

1 Dixon P, Peart E and Carr-Hill R (1999) *A Database of Examples of Consumer Involvement in Research.* University of York, York.

2 Entwistle VA, Renfrew MJ, Yearly S *et al.* (1998) Lay perspectives: advantages for health research. *BMJ.* **316**: 463–6.

3 Hanley B, Bradburn J, Gorin S *et al.* (2000) *Involving Consumers in Research and Development in the NHS.* Briefing notes for researchers. The Help for Health Trust, Winchester.

4 Walshe K and Ham C (1997) *Acting on the Evidence.* University of Birmingham, Birmingham.

Chapter 5

Vignettes from the literature

This chapter outlines some examples from the literature on lay involvement, and the action arising from lay involvement in research.

Early maps of lay involvement in NHS research and development

Oliver from the University of London provided an early map of examples and progress of lay involvement in NHS research and development.[1] Up until then the approaches had involved lay people in identifying research need and in the subsequent commissioning process. Oliver found lay contributions had given particular emphasis to information and support, whether this is in maternity care, cancer care, HIV prevention, participation in clinical trials or systematically reviewing evidence of effectiveness.[1] The difficulties Oliver identified nearly 10 years ago still exist and need attention today: identifying appropriate lay people to involve in research, the different skills of lay people, their lack of resources and support, and their need for time for thought and discussion with their peers have all posed problems. As to solutions, Oliver suggested various ways to dilute these problems including appropriate resourcing, training and support, and clarification of the role, nature and potential for lay involvement. Ahead of the times, Oliver concluded by asking for more evaluation of lay involvement in order to learn from others' efforts so far![1]

Lay involvement in research co-ordinating centres

Writing in the *BMJ*, Hanley and colleagues from the Consumers in NHS Research Support Unit sought to assess the extent to which consumers are involved in the work of clinical trial co-ordinating centres in the UK and the nature of consumers' involvement in randomised trials co-ordinated by these centres.[2] National surveys using structured questionnaires with some open-ended sections were used in this research project. Over one hundred (103) clinical trial co-ordinating centres in the UK were identified through a database assembled in 1997 by the NHS clinical trials adviser. Named contacts at 62 of the co-ordinating centres and investigators in 60 trials were identified as involving consumers.

Of the 62 eligible centres, 23 (37%) reported that consumers had already been involved in their work, and most respondents were positive about this involvement. Seventeen (27%) of the centres planned to involve consumers, 15 (24%) had no plans to involve consumers, and four of these considered lay involvement to be irrelevant.

Responses from investigators about the 48 individual trials were mostly positive, with respondents commenting that input from consumers had helped refine research questions, improve the quality of patient information, and make the trial more relevant to the needs of patients. Hanley and colleagues argue that consumer involvement in the design and conduct of controlled trials seems to be growing and seems to be welcomed by most researchers.[2] The authors go on to suggest that such involvement seems likely to improve the relevance to consumers of the questions addressed and the results obtained in controlled trials.

Lay involvement in needs-led research

Oliver and colleagues from the University of London sought to describe the methods used for involving consumers in a needs-led health research programme, and to discuss facilitators, barriers and goals.[3] They drew on the experience of campaigning, self-help and patients' representative groups, national charities, health information services, consumer researchers and journalists for various tasks. They explored consumer literature as a potential source for research questions, and as a route for disseminating research findings. A reflective approach included interviews with consumers, co-ordinating staff, external observers and other programme contributors, document analysis and multidisciplinary discussion (including consumers of course) amongst programme contributors.

When seeking research topics, Oliver and colleagues report that face-to-face discussion with a consumer group was more productive than scanning consumer research reports or contacting consumer health information services.[3] Consumers were willing and able to play active roles as panel members in refining and prioritising topics, and in commenting on research plans and reports. Training programmes for consumer involvement in service planning were readily adapted for a research programme. Challenges to be overcome were cultural divides, language barriers and a need for skills development amongst consumers and others.

Oliver and colleagues go on to submit that lay involvement in research highlighted a need for support and training for all contributors to the research programme.[3] They suggest that lay involvement benefited from the National Co-ordinating Centre for Health Technology Assessment (NCCHTA) staff being comfortable with innovation, participative development and team learning. Neither recruitment nor research capacity were insurmountable challenges according to Oliver and co-workers, but ongoing effort is required if lay involvement is to be sustained.

Meaningful participation in research process and outcomes

Ochocka and colleagues from the Centre for Research and Education in Human Services, analysed the process and outcomes of consumer/survivor researchers' involvement in a community mental health research project.[4] In this study the research roles and relationships were re-examined by both professional and consumer/survivor researchers. Ochocka and colleagues found that four values were central to the research process: consumer/survivor empowerment, supportive relationships, learning as an ongoing process, and social justice. The benefits of this value-driven approach were seen in terms of positive impacts on the lives of individual researchers and also in the quality of the research itself. Ochocka and colleagues suggest the importance of building relationships as a means to sharing power and knowledge among professional and consumer/survivor researchers.[4]

Professionals encouraging meaningful participation of select groups

How can professionals encourage meaningful participation of select groups of the population, e.g. individuals with mental retardation, in their research and training activities? Heller and colleagues sought to answer this question by interviewing 22 individuals.[5] These individuals had mental retardation as well as experience in research and training. The individuals had participated in various roles in research and training, but barriers to more meaningful involvement persisted and were not being adequately addressed. Heller and colleagues provided a set of still-usable guidelines for professionals to foster meaningful consumer involvement in their research and training activities.[5]

Lay involvement as voting members of scientific review panels

Andejeski and colleagues used cross-sectional analysis to evaluate the impact of having breast cancer survivors with advocacy experience participate as voting members of scientific review panels for proposals on breast cancer research.[6] In general, the voting patterns of breast cancer survivors were similar to those of scientists. Final proposal scores were the same as those that would have been obtained without consumer voting for 76.2% of the proposals, more favourable for 15.2% of the proposals, and less favourable for 8.6% of the proposals. For all but 13 proposals, the difference was ±0.1. Pre-panel opinions regarding consumer involvement were generally positive. Pre-panel and post-panel comparisons almost always showed that significantly greater proportions of participants had positive post-panel opinions than had negative post-panel opinions. Indeed Andejeski and colleagues found that having consumers on review panels was reported to be beneficial (83.9% and 98.2% for scientists and consumers, respectively) and to not have drawbacks (74.7% and 87.3%, respectively).[6]

Lay involvement as service users' advisory groups

Rhodes and colleagues looked at some of the issues raised by patients' involvement in the research process. They use the example of a service users' advisory group that was established as part of a diabetes evaluation project in the north of England.[7] Their main conclusions are:

- a precise role for the group should be specified at the outset
- genuine user involvement is needed

- wide and accurate representation of all relevant groups in society is essential
- researchers must approach users with open minds with a view to shared decision making rather than control.

Lay involvement of South Asian diabetic women who do not speak English

In late 2002 Rhodes and colleagues reported on a research advisory group project in Bradford for South Asian women with diabetes who do not speak English.[8] The following is an extract from their report:

> An evaluation of diabetes services was carried out in Bradford between 1999 and 2001. From the outset, it was agreed that local service users should be given an opportunity to contribute to the research process. Having ascertained the linguistic background of the women who showed an interest in attending, meetings were conducted in Punjabi by an Asian facilitator.
>
> Members of the Women's Advisory Group were recruited through a variety of methods: half through service providers (diabetes specialist nurses and GPs) and half through an Asian women's community centre and word-of-mouth. The first contact with the women was made by telephone by the facilitator, who explained the purpose and nature of the group and invited them to participate. Eight people, aged from early 40s to late 70s, agreed to take part (three refused on grounds of ill-health or prior commitment).
>
> Members of the group commented that the meetings held in the local hospital helped to make them feel that their views were valued. The women were offered lifts to and from the meetings: this seemed to give them confidence as they did not have to walk into the room on their own and could chat with the facilitator and other women in the car. The provision of transport and offer of token payments of £20 for each attendance were important factors in ensuring initial acceptance and continued commitment. With participants' agreement, meetings were taped, partially transcribed and translated.
>
> Some of the women were illiterate, yet were able to make a meaningful contribution to the research. They were able to comment on the relevance of interview questions and highlight issues that were important to them as a group and likely to be

important to other Asian people with diabetes. Personal experience can provide a valuable contribution to the research process, not least in the form of information sources and personal and community networks. Through participating in the group, members were able to move from the personal to the collective, to identify points of similarity and of difference through sharing their experiences with others, and to begin to think more strategically at the level of the group.

Benefits for the researchers of holding the groups included:

• helpful comments on research design and suggestions about recruitment of the interview sample, payment of interviewees, how to approach people, how to access 'hard to reach' groups, how to conduct interviews and content of interviews
• access to a range of different service users' views and experiences
• access to other networks
• promotion of goodwill towards the project in the wider community
• potential publicity about the project in the wider community
• promotion of greater understanding of research within the wider community
• practical help with the research, e.g. useful contacts and offers of help with interpreting and translation.

For the female participants, membership of the group provided an opportunity to:

• share information about services and treatments
• give each other advice
• learn about the research process
• offer and receive mutual support – particularly important for people living with a disease which can be both isolating and debilitating.

Lay involvement an organisational infrastructure

Stevens and colleagues from Sheffield reported on a project where they sought to overcome the challenges to lay involvement (they use the term 'consumers') in cancer research.[9] Three innovations were examined in detail:

1 How three open consumer conferences have increased awareness of research amongst service users (e.g. posters on current research being displayed for non-researchers).

2 The recruitment of consumers to sit on project steering groups and a committee that provides a strategic overview of current research.
3 The establishment of a consumer panel for research where reimbursed, trained consumers are able to provide a consumer perspective in a range of settings.

Stevens and colleagues argue against *ad hoc* single project lay involvement, and this suggests the need to build systems and procedures to improve and maintain lay involvement in research.[9]

Learning from a failed lay consultation

Graham and colleagues from the Australian National University, Canberra, sought to understand the barriers to obtaining input from consumers in developing public health research.[10] They employed an analysis of documentation of a failed attempt at consumer consultation. Whilst people are keen to be heard in the formulation of health research, competing demands and limited resources make it difficult for community groups to allocate scarce resources to consultation. Sometimes research issues may seem 'academic' and thus remote from the urgent priorities of the people with whom researchers wish to consult. Consultation may require more time than researchers on limited budgets can afford. Graham and colleagues rightly suggest that researchers and funding bodies will need to allocate resources to consumer consultation if it is to become the norm rather than the exception in public health research.[10]

Lay involvement in professional education, training and development

A variety of authors have looked at issues which arise when we look at incorporating users of services as part of the programmes for training professionals delivering the services. For example, Wood and Wilson-Barnett looked at the influence of user involvement on the learning of mental health nursing students.[11] Comparing two groups of students exposed to different amounts of user involvement during training, Wood and Wilson-Barnett used student surveys and classroom observations. They found that students with higher levels of exposure to user involvement had a more individualised approach to mental health assessment, showed greater empathy and used less jargon in mental health assessment.[11] A follow-up-study would, if conducted, seek to establish if these characteristics were carried into professional practice post-training.

Flanagan from the University of Leeds provides an innovative example of user and carer involvement in the design of continuing education and higher education in cancer care nursing within the University of Leeds School of Healthcare Studies.[12] On the basis that users of health services and their carers can contribute to the planning and delivery of professional education courses, Flanagan provides insight into the positive aspects and challenges presented by such involvement.

Lay involvement with users as peer supporters

Klein and colleagues used a pilot study of peer support in service use.[13] Whilst this may not be lay involvement in research in itself, it does raise some questions for subsequent research. Klein and colleagues looked at two different programmes (a case management-only programme compared to a case management and support from user–employees programme). Their pilot research found that users in contact with the peer support programme had fewer inpatient days, improved social functioning, and some improvements to their quality of life compared to the case management-only group. A follow-up study would help to establish if these results hold in a larger sample of people.

Lay involvement in guideline development

Bastian looks at consumer participation in guideline development.[14] Bastian argues that if consumer involvement is to successfully raise the standard of healthcare guidelines, then the standard of consumer participation itself needs to be raised. To do this a combination of three strategies is suggested: the involvement of an accountable consumer representative in group decision making on the guidelines; community consultations in developing guidelines; and making better use of the emerging literature describing people's experiences with guidelines.

Further vignettes of lay involvement from the literature

Lay members are also involved in other aspects of healthcare as the following examples clearly show. These examples suggest that certain lessons on involvement can be taken from others' experiences.

Lay involvement in health committees

From the Consumers for Ethics in Research Unit, University of North London, Hogg and Williamson attempted to understand the role of lay people as members of health committees.[15] They indicate that the term 'lay' is used loosely and the reasons for involving lay people are seldom clearly defined. They argue that the different roles that lay people play need to be explicitly defined in order for their contributions to be realised. Hogg and Williamson found that although lay members of health service committees are generally assumed to be working for patients' interests, some tended to support professionals' or managers' interests rather than patients' interests as patients would define them.

Lay involvement in primary care groups/trusts

According to a University of Bristol-led study, Rowe suggests that lay members of primary care groups and trusts are increasingly confident in their ability to influence decision making.[16] An earlier King's Fund report suggested that lay members of primary care groups were finding it difficult to ensure that patients' views are heard.

In a postal survey of all primary care groups in the South West region (response rate 76%), Rowe reveals in the *BMJ* that 69% of lay members reported that:

- they had either moderate or a lot of influence over decision making
- their influence has increased with time as a result of their contribution to the work of the group
- they have gained credibility and earned the board's respect for their skills and experience.

Their main contribution lies, according to Rowe, in fulfilling their responsibilities as corporate board members, although many have taken the lead in public engagement.

The remaining 31% of lay members reported either limited or very limited influence; this was not associated with age, sex, prior knowledge of the NHS, or extent of previous board experience. Rather, isolation as the lone lay voice, lack of time, and general practitioners' dominance of the primary care group's agenda and decision making were reported as key constraints.[16]

Such self-reports can always be criticised as lacking objectivity, Rowe suggests, but they do reflect the level of confidence that lay members have in their ability to influence decisions, which is likely to be reflected in their participation in decision making. Rowe suggests that the Bristol survey highlights that lay members have a dynamic and evolving role, their influence increasing with knowledge and experience and through successful interaction with other board members.[16] Where lay members have been able to contribute their skills, this has caused other board members to revise their views on the benefits of lay participation, which in time may foster a culture that supports wider public involvement in the work of primary care groups and trusts. The bottom line according to Rowe is this: 'Don't write lay members off too soon'.

Lay involvement and consulting the locals

Alborz and colleagues from the University of Manchester report on primary care groups and trusts (PCG/Ts)' consultations with local communities.[17] Using evidence from the National Tracker Survey, they assess how the PCG/Ts have informed and consulted local communities and the perceived impact of this consultation on decision making. The National Tracker Survey was a longitudinal survey of 72 (15%) of the PCG/Ts in England, data from telephone interviews with chairs and chief officers, and postal questionnaires to lay board members and representatives of Community Health Councils (CHCs). Eighty-one per cent of PCG/Ts had public involvement working groups. Methods of consulting the community included consulting CHCs (87%), holding public meetings (75%) and consulting local patient groups (67%). Only 31% of chairs felt they were effective at consulting.

Ninety-two per cent of CHC representatives attended all board meetings. Most CHC representatives reported that there had been little or no consultation with the CHC in areas such as commissioning, service development or clinical governance. Only 14% of CHC representatives rated PCG/T consultation with the public as effective. Eighty-seven per cent said that local communities were largely unaware of the existence of PCG/Ts, and 70% commented on the weaknesses in PCG/T efforts at public consultation. Public participation is being taken seriously by PCG/Ts, but most are struggling to develop effective ways of involving local communities. Efforts to involve the public may become little more than token gestures. The proposed abolition of CHCs may make it more difficult for PCG/Ts to obtain a lay perspective. Alborz and colleagues suggest that effective consultation requires the development of new methods and adequate resources, but a stronger lay voice in the governance structures of PCG/Ts is also needed.[17]

Consent to use information in electronic records for research purposes

Writing in the *BMJ* in February 2003, Willison and colleagues report on a study involving interviewing 17 patients and surveying 106 in family practice.[18] The idea was to assess patients' preferred method of consent for the use of information from electronic medical records for research purposes. Willison and colleagues found that most of the interviewees were willing to allow the use of their information for research purposes. However they also found that the majority preferred that consent was sought first either verbally or in writing. The seeking of consent to use data was considered by the patients as an important element of respect for the individual. Nevertheless little distinction was made by the patients between identifiable and anonomised data.

References

1 Oliver S (1996) The progress of lay involvement in the NHS research and development programme. *J Eval Clin Pract.* **2**: 273–80.

2 Hanley B, Truesdale A, King A *et al.* (2001) Involving consumers in designing, conducting, and interpreting randomised controlled trials: questionnaire survey. *BMJ.* **322**: 519–23 (Comment in *BMJ.* **7**: 48–9).

3 Oliver S, Milne R, Bradburn J *et al.* (2001) Involving consumers in a needs-led research programme: a pilot project. *Health Expect.* **4**: 18–28 (Comment in *Health Expect.* **4**: 1).

4 Ochocka J, Janzen R and Nelson G (2002) Sharing power and knowledge: professional and mental health consumer/survivor researchers working

together in a participatory action research project. *Psychiatr Rehabil J.* **25**: 379–87.

5 Heller T, Pederson EL and Miller AB (1996) Guidelines from the consumer: improving consumer involvement in research and training for persons with mental retardation. *Ment Retard.* **34**: 141–8.

6 Andejeski Y, Bisceglio IT, Dickersin K *et al.* (2002) Quantitative impact of including consumers in the scientific review of breast cancer research proposals. *J Womens Health Gend Based Med.* **11**: 379–88.

7 Rhodes P, Nocon A, Wright J *et al.* (2001) Involving patients in research: setting up a service users' advisory group. *J Manag Med.* **15**: 167–71.

8 Rhodes P, Nocon A, Booth M *et al.* (2002) A research advisory group for South Asian women with diabetes who do not speak English. *Consumers in NHS Research News.*

9 Stevens T, Wilde D, Hunt J *et al.* (2003) Overcoming the challenges to consumer involvement in cancer research. *Health Expect.* **6**: 81–8.

10 Graham J, Broom D and Whittaker A (2001) Consulting about consulting: challenges to effective consulting about public health research. *Health Expect.* **4**: 209–12.

11 Wood J and Wilson-Barnett J (1999) The influence of user involvement on the learning of mental health nursing students. *Nurs Times Res.* **4**: 257–70.

12 Flanagan J (1999) Public participation in the design of educational programmes for cancer nurses: a case report. *Eur J Cancer Care.* **8**: 107–12.

13 Klein AR, Cnaan RA and Whitecraft J (1998) Significance of peer support with dually diagnosed clients: findings from a pilot study. *Res Soc Work Practice.* **8**: 529–51.

14 Bastian H (1996) Raising the standard: practice guidelines and consumer participation. *Int J Qual Health Care.* **8**: 485–90.

15 Hogg C and Williamson C (2001) Whose interests do lay people represent? Towards an understanding of the role of lay people as members of committees. *Health Expect.* **4**: 2–9.

16 Rowe R (2001) Lay members can contribute much in primary care groups. *BMJ.* **323**: 167.

17 Alborz A, Wilkin D and Smith K (2002) Are primary care groups and trusts consulting local communities? *Health Soc Care Community.* **10**: 20–8.

18 Willison DJ, Keshavjee K, Nair K *et al.* (2003) Patients' consent preferences for research uses of information in electronic medical records: interview and survey data. *BMJ.* **326**: 373–6.

Further reading

- Desario J and Langton S (1987) *Citizen Participation in Public Decision Making.* Greenwood Press, New York.
- Dunkerley D and Glasner P (1998) Empowering the public? Citizens' juries and the new genetic technologies. *Crit Public Health.* **8**: 181–92.
- Earl-Slater A (2002) *The Handbook of Clinical Trials and Other Research.* Radcliffe Medical Press, Oxford.
- Hanley B (1999) Research and development in the NHS: how can you make a difference? *Health Expect.* **2**: 72.
- Mandl KD, Szolovits P, Kohane IS *et al.* (2001) Public standards and patients' control: how to keep electronic medical records accessible but private. *BMJ.* **322**: 283–7.
- Rhodes P, Nocon A, Booth M *et al.* (2001) A users' advisory group in practice. *Consumers in NHS Research News,* Autumn: **6**.
- Upshur RE, Morin B and Goel V (2001) The privacy paradox: laying Orwell's ghost to rest. *CMAJ.* **165**: 307–9.

Chapter 6

Wider issues in lay involvement

It can be argued that public confidence in health research has been eroded in recent years and the erosion cannot be allowed to continue. Whilst we all want more effective and efficient healthcare, we also expect more accountability, greater transparency and increased due process (people explaining their decisions and providing the evidence base to justify them) as to what is being researched, with what resources, to what time scale, why, and with what impact. As a consequence we may have a new humility amongst some researchers and a new assertiveness amongst the public. Today, more than ever before, the public expects not merely to know what is going on, but to be consulted and listened to. Researchers must link their research arenas and make stronger and longer connections with their wider communities and the public, from developing research topics through to evaluation and dissemination.

How then can you open opportunities for wider public engagement which simultaneously achieve these ends and maintain high-quality relevant research? Some lessons and techniques can and should be learnt from the evidence of the Select Committee on Science and Technology:[1]

- consultations at national level
- consultations at local level
- deliberative polling
- standing consultative panels
- focus groups
- citizens' juries
- lay involvement in inspections
- consensus conferences
- stakeholder dialogues
- Internet dialogues
- foresight.

Whilst some of these are only relevant for national research projects, there is no reason why they cannot be linked into local networks. In September 2001, the Department of Health set out its proposals for implementing their vision of a patient-centred NHS.[2] This was outlined in *The NHS Plan*,[3] and built on the provisions in the Health and Social Care Act 2001. The Department of Health's proposals included:

- the introduction of Patient Advocacy and Liaison Services (PALS) – providing information and on-the-spot help – in every trust
- providing a locally-based Independent Complaints Advocacy Service (ICAS) in England, operating to core standards
- introducing patients' forums in every trust, to bring the patient's perspective in trust management decision making. These forums would also be able to elect one of their members to sit on the trust board as a non-executive director
- extending Local Authority Overview and Scrutiny Committees (LAOSC) powers to scrutinise local health services and to call NHS managers to account
- setting up a 'voice' in every strategic health authority area – a professional group acting as a local resource for helping communities
- setting up a new national patients' body to set standards and provide training, and to monitor the new arrangements.

Whilst these are Department of Health proposals, here are some ideas on how they could be used to build networks that include research and lay involvement. Each proposal has an opportunity to help improve research, for example:

- PALS can hold information on what research is taking place in the trust, and share information about successful and unsuccessful lay involvement in local research
- patients' forums can cover topics such as lay member recruitment, induction and training, local research management, local research projects, research training and research dissemination
- LAOSCs can cover the management and progress of research in the trust
- 'voices' can do for the strategic health authority what patients' forums do for the trust
- standards can be set on lay member recruitment, training, retention, and rewards.

In what follows I provide engaging examples beyond healthcare. It always pays to look for lessons and illustrations beyond your own immediate environment.

Consultations at national level

Recall that I mentioned the NICE and MRC exercises earlier. Now I move onto other examples. Although involving only a small number of people the Government's Public Consultation on the Biosciences was considered time-consuming and expensive. Furthermore, the workshops were open to the charge of being directed by the organisers rather than the lay participants. However, there is a view that the lay participants were engaged by the issues, and developed 'rich understandings' as the workshops proceeded. Indeed, participants themselves rated the process highly, and were proud to take part. How the Government takes the 'rich understanding' forward remains to be seen.

The Wellcome Trust has been holding a series of national consultations on biomedical topics in recent years, as part of its Medicine in Society programme. These included public perspectives on human cloning and public attitudes to databases of human biological samples.

Consultations at local level

An application for a new energy-from-waste incinerator in Portsmouth failed to be accepted by the Hampshire County Council. The incinerator had been identified as the 'best practical environmental option', and some consultation had taken place. However local pressure groups and Portsmouth City Council together defeated the plan. According to the Select Committee reports 'neither the developer nor the county council had made a full effort to listen to people's views and to take them on board during the development of the proposal'. In an effort to avoid repeating the same mistake twice, the county council launched (in 1993) an elaborate two-year public consultation consisting of:

- a community advisory forum for each of three areas, with an independent chairman and members representing a range of community interests
- a public information programme
- focus groups consisting of members of the public chosen at random
- a questionnaire survey.

The advisory forums reached consensus on a need for an integrated strategy for waste management (to include energy-from-waste incineration). In 1995 the council produced a strategy, which was the subject of further consultation before being finalised in 1996. The whole exercise involved genuine public consultation. Accordingly:

> The county council gained an understanding that public responses to proposals for waste disposal facilities which had previously been categorised as not in my back yard (NIMBY)

should not be dismissed as irrational, subjective and based on self-interest, but masked issues that had to be addressed about inequities in risk-sharing and lack of trust in decision takers.

Professor Roland Clift commented that the consultation:

got into the public debate the idea that doing nothing was not an option. That immediately focuses the deliberative process on finding an outcome rather than merely accepting or rejecting a solution which is imposed by somebody else.[1]

Deliberative polling

In a deliberative poll, a large representative group of perhaps, say, several hundred people conducts a debate on an issue. The group is polled on the issue before and after the debate. Generally a deliberative poll is a fairly crude, one-off market research type of exercise with a typical poll costing around £20 000–25 000.

Standing consultative panels

The UK is reputed to be the first country in the world to set up a standing consultative panel at national level. The so-called People's Panel consists of 5000 members of the public, selected at random from across the UK, available as a basis for market research, quantitative and qualitative research and consultation. The People's Panel was set up in 1998 by Market and Opinion Research International (MORI) and Birmingham University for the Cabinet Office. Its main objective is to trace and record levels of satisfaction with public services, but it is also available for other purposes. For instance, it has been used in the public consultation on the biosciences.

It is possible to maintain a panel with a more limited remit. For example, the Wellcome Trust has a consultative panel on gene therapy.

Focus groups

Focus groups are used widely in commercial market research and increasingly in some academic research (e.g. sociology). Typically, a group of around 10–20 people, preferably broadly representative of the population being studied, is invited to discuss the issue of concern. Focus groups are usually guided by a trained facilitator working to a pre-designed discussion protocol. The focused discussion may last up to two to four hours. The group is not required to reach any conclusions, but the contents of discussion are studied for what they may reveal about understandings, attitudes, language and values, with respect to the issue. Focus groups may also help to identify the factors that shape attitudes and responses, including trust.

Citizens' juries

A citizens' jury often involves a relatively small group of lay participants (say 10–20) receiving, questioning, discussing and evaluating presentations by experts on a particular issue, usually over one or two days. At the end, the group is invited to make recommendations. Citizens' juries have been widely used for market research by local authorities, government agencies, policy researchers and consultants, on various issues. For example in 1997, the Welsh Institute for Health and Social Care ran a citizens' jury on genetic testing for common disorders; and the Economic and Social Research Council (ESRC) ran one on the European Union (EU) single market, as an experiment in dissemination of social science research, in the same year.

A citizens' jury is a less ambitious, and usually a cheaper exercise than a consensus conference. It is nevertheless a demanding process, and requires professional management and analysis. One might cost around £15 000–25 000.

Lay involvement in inspections

The following is an abstract from the Social Services Inspectorate (SSI).

> The SSI recruits and trains volunteers to work with its full-time professional inspectors to help inspect the way social service departments and independent agencies provide services for children, older people and people with disabilities. These volunteers are known in the SSI world as lay assessors and are drawn from various walks of life.
>
> As part of a team of specialists, the volunteers are fully involved in promoting good quality services and commenting

on the effectiveness and efficiency of the personal social services and ensuring the safety and wellbeing of the people who use them. Involving lay people in this way helps our inspections benefit from fresh perspectives, independence of viewpoint and diverse experiences of life and work.

Each volunteer is usually needed for up to two or three inspections a year and for up to 10 days for each inspection. This includes pre-inspection planning, inspection visits, and post-visit evaluation and reporting. People who can offer more or less time than this are welcome.

This is a voluntary role but car mileage and other out-of-pocket expenses are met. The area of operation is negotiable but most volunteers operate within their home region. Volunteers do not work in the local authority where they live.

Academic or occupation background is not important although all volunteers need to be observant, methodical and able to represent and support their views.

People who have experience of using social services, or who have experience as carers are welcome, so are people who have other kinds of experience, for example, in business, education or the voluntary sector. Applications from younger people and those from ethnic minority backgrounds are particularly welcome, as these groups are under-represented among current lay volunteers.

People who have a working background in health or personal social services are not eligible.

Everyone recruited is given training and appointments are usually for three years.

If you are interested in finding out more (e.g. if your research is about facilitating hospital discharge or care in the community) contact the Inspection Resource Group of the Social Service Inspectorate, Department of Health, London.

Consensus conferences

A typical consensus conference includes a balanced sample of around 10–20 lay volunteers. The group initially meets in private, to discuss the issue and to decide the key questions. There is then a public phase, lasting perhaps two to three days, during which the group hears and interrogates expert witnesses, and draws up a report.

The Danish Board of Technology held a consensus conference on the acceptability of irradiated food. The conference was established to help to inform policy and engage the public (including the media). Information from the irradiated food conference enabled the Danish Parliament to judge *correctly* that the public would not accept irradiation of food, whereas according to the Select Committee on Science and Technology, the UK Advisory Committee on Novel Foods and Processes judged *incorrectly* that the UK public would accept such food. Denmark has also held consensus conferences on gene technology, mapping the human genome, and IT in transport.

An early consensus conference in the UK was held in 1994, on the subject of plant biotechnology, i.e. genetically modified (GM) crops. Organised by the Biotechnology and Biological Sciences Research Council (BBSRC) and the Science Museum, the event itself was reckoned to have gone well, and according to reports in the Select Committee of Science and Technology 'it generated considerable interest and influenced some government departments and Members of Parliament [MPs]'. In fact it had no visible impact on policy.

Stakeholder dialogues

An unpalatable term to some of course, a 'stakeholder dialogue' is a consultation restricted to those who have, or who express, an interest in the subject matter. It is more than market research or public relations (PR), but less than a public consultation, which would have to include those who, at least to start with, were not at all interested. The Shell UK Exploration and Production 'Brent Spar' story is now a classic text book case study of stakeholder dialogues being used after problems were encountered relating to the company's plans to dispose of the Brent Spar offshore installation. In response, Shell engaged the Environment Council, a registered charity, to design and run a consultation process. From a list of 500 interested parties, the council selected groups to attend meetings held in London, Copenhagen, Rotterdam and Hamburg. At initial meetings in each place, the company posed the following question: 'What criteria would you use to select a shortlist of options to consider?' In the light of the answers, the company drew up a shortlist, and invited contractors to make proposals, which were made public. At further meetings, the company invited stakeholders to place values on the various environmental and safety factors involved.

At all these meetings, the Environment Council provided chairmen; Shell's role was simply to provide necessary information, and then sit back and listen. There was no requirement to reach a consensus and of course responsibility for making decisions remained with the company and the Government. Stakeholder dialogues are only important if they are listened to and the information is used to help formulate transparent decisions.

According to Professor Conway's testimony in the Select Committee on Science and Technology report,[1] the directors of Monsanto should be urged to engage in stakeholder dialogues (is it too late?). Professor Conway called for a global public dialogue – which will involve everyone on an equal footing – the seed companies, consumer groups, environmental groups, independent scientists and representatives of governments.[2] Conway proposed the following elements:

- a list of all the possible areas of risk and of benefit and an attempt to prioritise them
- the creation of a range of forums for discussion, including use of the Internet
- a truly impartial public education effort based on the global list of risks and benefits
- concessions on the part of Monsanto
- full disclosure and transparency of evidence, materials and decisions
- respecting the process.

Internet dialogues

The Internet can be used to enable consultation, in any of the modes described above. It can also be used to escape from the confines of 'place'. An Internet dialogue may be closed to a selected list of participants; or it may be open to anyone with Internet access. As access increases, Internet dialogues are becoming an increasingly powerful tool for consultation and contribution.

Internet dialogues are cheap and easy to run for anyone with the necessary technology. The Internet is a popular medium; it enables a lot of responses to be collected quickly. It combines the advantages of rapid exchange of ideas (brainstorming) with a complete record. But participation is too often self-selecting and unrepresentative and the anonymity of the Internet may encourage impulsive rather than considered responses. The provenance of information may be difficult to weigh and this militates against confidence. The quality of information and debate on the Internet may be low, and participants may have little confidence that views expressed this way make a difference. These problems can be diminished if the Internet dialogue facilitator has a sufficiently high profile, and the participants have, and stick to, a clear set of principles.

Foresight (informed speculation)

The purpose of a foresight exercise is usually to:

- provide people with a coherent view as to what the future will look like
- inform people about change
- prepare them for change
- help them to cope with change.

Foresight programmes can be of various formats as above including *ad hoc* or standing groups meeting periodically to reflect on new information and understanding. It is usually an ambitious and speculative programme but has some value in terms of planning ahead for research lines and different scenarios in terms of the dissemination of research findings and prospects for implementing change.

References

1   Select Committee on Science and Technology (2000) Third Report. Science and Society. Select Committee on Science and Technology, London.
2   Department of Health (2001) *Involving Patients and the Public in Healthcare: a discussion document*. DoH, London.
3   Department of Health (2001) *The NHS Plan: a plan for investment, a plan for reform*. DoH, London.

Further reading

- Earl-Slater A (2002) *The Handbook of Clinical Trials and Other Research*. Radcliffe Medical Press, Oxford.

Chapter 7

Research methods

This chapter on research methods has the following aims:

- to provide vignettes on various methods used for lay involvement
- to promote the idea of more than one method being available
- to offer ideas that multiple strategies may be necessary in the research
- to help ensure some attention is paid to research methods
- to identify discussion points about how everyone in your research team is going to learn about the research methods and their rationale in the project.

Table 7.1 outlines the different methods used to collect data in various research projects.

Table 7.2 provides an indication of the methods that were used by lay members to collect data in various projects.

The rest of this chapter goes on to outline some of the key aspects of different research methods. Some of this has been highlighted earlier, but if lay members are to be involved in your research and in collecting information, then an acquaintance with some of the methods employed is required. For a wider and deeper discourse on research methods then *The Handbook of Clinical Trials and Other Research*[1] is a good contemporary source of advice, information, insight and inspiration.

Documentary analysis

Documentary analysis is the study of documents in terms of their:

- source
- date
- target audience
- content
- logic
- links with other relevant evidence
- strengths and weaknesses.

Table 7.1: Main research designs in the project

Title of topic	Main research design in the project
Cancer voices	• Action research
Patient and carer views of stroke services	• Study of views/experiences
A randomised controlled trial to evaluate the benefit of a new information leaflet for parents of children hospitalised with benign febrile convulsions	• Randomised controlled trial • Comparison of effects of new leaflet with the previous written information • Evaluation
A large randomised long-term assessment of the relative cost-effectiveness of surgery for Parkinson's disease	• Randomised controlled trial
Survey of views of people affected by motor neurone disease on the only drug treatment (then) available: riluzole	• Study of views/experiences
Evaluating the multiple sclerosis (MS) specialist nurse: a review and development of the role	• Action research • Case study • Evaluation • Study of views/experiences
Torbay Healthy Housing Group: Watcombe Project	• Randomised controlled trial
Medication education	• Evaluation
Befriending: more than just finding friends?	• Evaluation • Study of views/experiences
Practice guidelines for primary healthcare teams to meet South Asian Carers' needs	• Systematic review • Qualitative methods
What happens to people with severe aphasia?	• Action research • Study of views/experiences • Ethnography
Collaborative studies on health service and quality of life in people with learning disability	• Cohort study • Evaluation • Study of views/experiences • Systematic review
Joint replacement	• Case study • Cohort study • Evaluation • Randomised controlled trial • Study of views/experiences • Systematic review
Cognitive remediation: a randomised controlled trial	• Randomised controlled trial
People's experiences of screening assessment by nurses in a community mental health team	• Study of views/experiences
Disability equipment evaluations	• Evaluation • Study of views/experiences
Cochrane skin group	• Systematic review
Developing and evaluating best practice for user involvement in cancer services	• Study of views/experiences

Table 7.2: Examples of methods used by lay members to collect data in projects

Title of topic	Involvement methods employed
Cancer voices	• Focus groups • Questionnaire survey
Patient and carer views of stroke services	• Focus groups
A randomised controlled trial to evaluate the benefit of a new information leaflet for parents of children hospitalised with benign febrile convulsions	• Interviews • Questionnaire survey
A large randomised long-term assessment of the relative cost-effectiveness of surgery for Parkinson's disease	• Outcome measures
Survey of views of people affected by motor neurone disease on the only drug treatment (then) available: riluzole	• Interviews • Questionnaire survey
Evaluating the multiple sclerosis (MS) specialist nurse: a review and development of the role	• Documentary analysis • Focus groups • Interviews • Questionnaire survey • Observation • Outcome measures
Torbay Healthy Housing Group: Watcombe Project	• Interviews • Questionnaire survey • Various environmental measures
Medication education	• Outcome measures
Befriending: more than just finding friends?	• Documentary analysis • Interviews
Practice guidelines for primary healthcare teams to meet South Asian Carers' needs	• Focus groups • Interviews
What happens to people with severe aphasia?	• Documentary analysis • Interviews • Questionnaire survey • Observation • Ethnographic evidence
Collaborative studies on health service and quality of life in people with learning disability	• Documentary analysis • Focus groups • Interviews • Questionnaire survey • Observation • Outcome measures
Joint replacement	• Focus groups • Interviews • Questionnaire survey
Cognitive remediation: a randomised controlled trial	• Interviews • Outcome measures
People's experiences of screening assessment by nurses in a community mental health team	• Interviews
Disability equipment evaluations	• Focus groups • Interviews • Questionnaire survey • Cross-over trials
Cochrane skin group	• Documentary analysis • Focus groups
Developing and evaluating best practice for user involvement in cancer services	• Focus groups • Interviews • Questionnaire survey

Sources of documents include publications by government, regulatory bodies, companies, individuals, academic establishments, professional bodies, patient advocacy groups, charitable bodies, or proceedings of conferences or symposia, research protocols or research governance reports.

The documents may or may not be in the public domain.

Advantages of documentary research and analysis include their:

- non-reactivity with the investigator
- permanence of record
- accessibility (in general).

Disadvantages of documentary analysis include:

- questions over authenticity and accuracy
- questions in interpretation
- questions of completeness
- no document is a complete and accurate representation of the phenomenon of interest
- few documents indicate their process of construction
- few documents indicate their set of assumptions
- documents are time-dependent and often go out of date.

Observational study

An observational study is a method of assessment that is carried out by an observer who, at best, identifies, observes, records, classifies and analyses relevant information in a study without interfering with the course of events. An observational study must have a clear objective. To do an observation that has no clear objective is a waste of everyone's time and resources: it is futile and pointless.

Whilst having a clear objective is paramount in observation analysis, nothing can be gained if there is no method of recording events, people and time scales involved, and resources involved. Careful and judicious thought therefore has to be made in advance of the observation as to what will be recorded, by whom, where, why and when. Attention also has to be focused on issues relating to confidentiality and ethics. The first few observations may form part of a pilot exercise, testing what can be recorded. It has also been the case that information and experience from some pilot observations have in fact changed the original question under investigation. Subsequent observations then build on the pilot by using, say, a more structured systematic format, in a sense building a virtuous cycle of observation and analysis.

Cohort study

A cohort study is an observational study of a particular group over a period of time.

- A retrospective cohort study looks back over time e.g. at all those who had antithrombotic treatment for atrial fibrillation, or all those who had paediatric cardiac surgery.
  - Ely and colleagues sought to determine if there was any evidence that greater medical knowledge was associated with increased malpractice claims.[2] They used a cohort study linking data from medical directories and family practice certification examination scores with medical malpractice insurance claims.
  - In a five-year retrospective cohort study of 138 acute care hospitals, Glasgow and colleagues sought to determine if higher hospital volume was associated with lower operative mortality and shorter length of stay after hepatic resection.[3]
  - Reid and colleagues reported on a retrospective cohort study of medically unexplained symptoms in frequent attenders of secondary healthcare.[4]
- A prospective cohort study looks forward over time e.g. to determine how many people with a specified risk factor go on to develop the disease of interest.
  - Doll and colleagues used a prospective study of 34 439 male British doctors to assess the possible association between smoking and dementia.[5]
  - Evans and colleagues used a cohort study to identify and examine pregnant women's depression during pregnancy and after childbirth.[6]

Advantages of cohort studies include that:

- they are relatively cheaper to carry out than a clinical trial
- they may be done more quickly than a clinical trial
- they can, to an extent, be used to examine cause and effect
- they follow a select group over a period of time.

Some of the disadvantages of cohort studies are that:

- they do not involve a control group
- they can be prone to loss of study subjects over time
- they may not be generalisable.

Randomised controlled trial

A randomised controlled trial is a clinical trial where:

- patients are randomly allocated to different regimens in the trial
- some patients get the regimen of prime interest (e.g. a new drug)
- other patients get another regimen – the controls (e.g. 'usual care' or placebo).

This design allows the assessment of the relative effectiveness of the different regimens by comparing processes, event rates and outcomes.

Such a trial could include medicines, surgery, technology, exercise, diet, systems of organisation, grades of staff used, information offered and educational efforts. There are few limits to what can be included in a randomised controlled trial.

As an example of a published randomised controlled trial, Freemantle and colleagues evaluated the effectiveness and efficiency of visits by trained pharmacists in delivering messages to general practitioners.[7] The pharmacists received special training and the messages were derived from four evidence-based clinical practice guidelines.

Montgomery and colleagues ran a randomised controlled trial to evaluate a computer-based clinical decision support system and risk chart for management of hypertension in primary care.[8]

In general, randomised controlled trials are thought to offer the best methods to determine the merits of different regimens. Some argue that they are the 'gold standard' method of providing information of the relative merits of interventions. Yet the quality of randomised controlled trials can and has been questioned (see later sections in this book on the advantages and disadvantages of evidence from formal research, barriers to using the evidence in practice, and hierarchies of the evidence).

Systematic review

A systematic review is an approach of capturing and assessing the evidence by some systematic method, where all the components of the approach and the assessment are made explicit and documented.

Some examples of components include:

- a clear research question
- where the researchers looked for information (e.g. Medline, Controlled Trials, Embase, NHS National Research Register)

- what criteria they used to select the evidence
- what criteria they used to discard particular pieces of evidence
- how the evidence was collated
- how the key messages were derived.

Systematic reviews are based on several premises:

- large quantities of information must be made into smaller pieces for consumption
- such reviews integrate critical pieces of available information
- a review is usually quicker and less expensive than a new study
- the generalisability of the evidence can be established
- the consistency of relationships can be established
- inconsistencies in the evidence can be determined
- gaps in the evidence can be identified
- increases in the statistical power of studies can be achieved.

Focus group

A focus group is essentially a group of individuals that are brought together for a period of time to focus on a particular issue or set of issues. Focus groups have been used to test out ideas and draft plans, to draw out the views and opinions, experiences and expectations of certain people when expressed in a group situation. Focus groups can be as small as four people and some have been as large as 100. However, 100 is probably too large for one group – it may be more effective and more efficient to have 10 groups of 10 people, or groups of 10–15, than one big group of 100.

The focus group must have a purpose and a set of working principles. These must be explicit and understood by all involved in the research. Some of the best focus groups I have come across have been run like the very best business meetings.

Good practice suggests that the best focus groups:

- have a clear objective
- have a clear and consistent set of applicable principles
- have a predefined time scale
- are well managed
- accurately record progress, events and decisions
- are non-threatening to any individual or subgroups of individuals involved
- provide a safe environment in which to share thoughts, feelings and impressions

- have a clearly defined end-point
- know at the outset what will be done with the information gathered.

Unless you want to be involved in one that has a broad and sweeping remit, focus groups do well when they are run with professionalism and a liberal use of open questions. Depth may be more important than breadth in some focus groups. So you need to know the purpose and principles of the focus group before you get involved. If it has no clear purpose or set of principles do not get involved and do not accept its findings (if they are ever presented or published in a wide domain beyond the group and its sponsors that is).

Weaknesses of the focus groups include their possible unrepresentativeness and that of the dominance of views by certain members of the group. Great emphasis is therefore placed on the focus group facilitator to dilute and pre-empt dominance.

There is also the fear factor that may paralyse some valuable contributions if you ever feel that you may be 'tainted' by holding or expressing certain views in the focus group. Careful planning and leadership from the group's facilitator or manager should dilute these weaknesses. Nevertheless certain characters may emerge in focus groups as in other groups of people. These should not be frowned upon as they can enrich the group discussion and may better represent how the topic under focus will be greeted in a wider community. Diversity is taken to be a strength if, and only if, it is managed efficiently and effectively. Box 7.1 shows certain characters in groups.

In some cases focus groups have been used in a mechanical manner to give the members of the group, and those beyond, an impression of the researchers 'listening' to their views and feelings.

Other pitfalls of focus groups are that they can:

- be used when one cannot think of anything else to do
- be badly managed
- have no particular points of focus
- be too few in number in terms of members
- be too big or too small in size
- be used when far too much is attempted in any one group session
- have not enough flexibility or latitude (whilst there may be a plan or map for the group you do not always, if ever, know in advance all that is going to come up in the group discussions)
- fail to inform the moderator or manager of the true purpose of the group
- use amateur or inappropriate moderators or managers
- use moderators or managers with vested interests in the topic being focused on.

Box 7.1: Characters in groups

Adopters
Agent provocateurs
Agony aunts and uncles
Complicators
Distractors
Dominators
Early adopters
Emotionalists
Explicators
Fragmenters
Gangs and factions
Innovators
Integrators
Investigators
Laggards
Late gadflies
Leaders
Passengers
Persuaders
Prophets of doom
Questioners
Self-styled captains of good news
Simplifiers
Soothsayers
Speculators
Submissives
Supporters
Visionaries
Wanderers
Witherers

Delphi technique

The Delphi technique is one of the qualitative research techniques that has been employed to engage and extract people's views, knowledge, understanding, articulation, feelings, opinions, language, and perspectives.

Generally in a Delphi technique, a collection of individuals is used to elicit viewpoints on a particular issue. The viewpoints could be on patient inclusion and exclusion criteria in a trial, what kind of trial to set up, how and what to measure in the research, the duration of the study, the importance of the results and how to manage change in light of the results.

The viewpoints have traditionally been obtained via mail or telephone, but increasingly Delphi techniques on the Internet (e.g. email) are being used. Under the Delphi technique the individuals may not know who has said what about a topic and the individuals do not meet others to discuss the issues under question. Properly managed, there are minimal opportunities for any one person's judgement to be influenced by any other. The standpoints of individuals are then gathered up and aggregated. This aggregate picture is then circulated to the individuals, and by an iterative process, areas of agreement and disagreement are determined. This can be considered the first round of the Delphi technique. Subsequent rounds, where the individuals are still kept separate, may be carried out. In subsequent rounds the aggregated, but not individual, views are usually circulated for comment and reflection.

The number of rounds in a Delphi exercise depends on factors such as the:

- primary objective of the exercise
- quality of information gained in the first round of using the technique
- probability of yielding more quality information and insight by conducting another round
- management efficiency
- analytical expertise
- risk of losing the goodwill or the participants
- pressures of time
- costs of conducting another round.

Questions that naturally arise with Delphi techniques are:

- who to include
- how to include them
- how to keep them distant from group pressures
- the topic for consideration
- how to collate the answers
- how to manage and moderate the process
- the time scales involved
- the internal rewards to those participating
- the external rewards that can be had from such an exercise to others beyond the participants, facilitators, sponsors or managers
- how many rounds to do

- whether the primary question changes in light of the information and views presented in each round (good quality Delphi techniques stick to one primary question but may supplement this with others as more rounds are undertaken – the risk being the prospect of identifying individuals or making individuals do more than was initially agreed)
- what to do with the information harvested.

For those who are interested in this angle, the word Delphi, in the classic history of mythology, was a small town in Phocis, the Pytho of Homer, celebrated for its oracle Apollo. Apollo was the god of prophecy.

Interviews

Interviews are one of the ways of collecting information you need and, as seen in Table 7.2, they have been used in projects with lay involvement. Interviews can be carried out over the telephone, by email, or most commonly face-to-face. Before an interview is conducted you need to set out the objectives. Interviews can be structured, semi-structured or what is called informal/unstructured. In a structured interview there is a set list of questions and the interviewer asks all these questions in the order as they are set out. If the interviewer is allowed some discretion or there is some flexibility within the framework then I call this a semi-structured interview. If there is no set of questions or no set order, then I call these informal or unstructured interviews. In the informal interviews the interviewer may have some themes to cover, can follow up unpredictable responses and use prompts to elicit further information. Informal interviews are usually used when you want to dig deeper into an issue, whereas formal structured interviews are usually used when you want to gather information from a relatively large number of people. The more standard the interview schedule the easier it is to collect and analyse the information (but this depends on the types of questions so it is worth reading the entry on questionnaires as well). Whatever form you adopt, the interview schedule should fulfil the study's objectives and build respondents' interest in your research. Interviews do not need a high literacy rate for respondents to be in a safe and comfortable position to be able to answer the questions.

Interviews can gain a better response rate and explore issues in a wider and deeper manner than questionnaires. Face-to-face interviews can build trust and confidence – especially important if you are going to come back to the interviewee later in the research project. Rather complex issues can be addressed, responses can be validated and prompts and visual aids can be used where necessary.

The interviewer's dress, timing, sex, age, mannerisms, ethnicity, speech, and the time and place of interview may all affect the responses. For instance a 'white-coat' may suggest 'authority and clinics', a business suit may be seen as 'managerial' and children, for instance, may respond differently to an interviewer in more casual dress than one in a suit or white-coat. Interviews are usually more time consuming and more expensive than questionnaires.

Some ethical issues surrounding interviewing exist (and of course these apply to questionnaires and other forms of research). In summary these are:

- voluntary participation – no one should be coerced into participating
- informed consent – potential candidates should be fully informed of the research
- risk of harm – no harm should come to those that do or do not participate
- confidentiality – respondents should be guaranteed confidentiality and told who will analyse the data, and how it will be used
- anonymity – participants should be told about the research project's arrangement for anonymity
- compensation for helping with the research (e.g. £10 to a charity of their choice).

Some practical issues surrounding interviewing need you and your research team's careful thought:

- sample selection (who do you interview and how were they chosen?)
- how to interview (face-to-face, telephone, other)
- who should interview (e.g. one of the research team, or an independent expert in interviewing)?
- what type of questions will be asked?
- are there any language issues – if so how will they be dealt with?
- introduction to the topic (tell participants why you are interviewing them)
- length of interview
- topics in the interview (does the interviewee need to know in advance what the themes are that will be coming up in the interview?)
- time and location of interview
- recording information and dealing with bias
- interviewer's skills (e.g. preparedness, decorum, politeness, attentiveness, responsiveness, organisation, sociability, listening skills, competence in prompting, and experience: do they need 'skilling up'?)
- piloting the interview (a quick exercise to see what works and what doesn't)

- balancing professionalism and efficiency without being overly friendly or seeking affinity in the interview
- ethical issues (see above)
- what will be done with the information?
- sponsorship – who is paying for it and why, has it influenced the research question and methods?
- resource issues – e.g. costs, training, facilities, materials, time, personnel
- closing the interview – what happens next?
- feedback – what will the lay person receive for their participation in the interview and when?

Interviewing has many pitfalls and whilst there is no comprehensive evidence showing how common certain pitfalls are, a list of possible pitfalls would help when designing an interview schedule, conducting an interview, and in interpreting results from an interview. Box 7.2 introduces a list of 21 pitfalls in interviewing that you and everyone in your research team need to be aware of.

Questionnaires

Questionnaires have long been used in health research and their merits are always under investigation. The key issues in questionnaires that you and your research team have to tackle are:

- piloting the questionnaire
- who to ask?
- what to ask?
- how to get their response
- the choice of wording (clear, unambiguous, jargon and cliché free)
- the type of questions
- the response format
- the sequence and length of questions
- presentation
- what to do with the results
- how to get sufficient responses (make the questions salient).

Type of questions

There are various ways to decide on types of questions and these need attention in the research especially in interviewing and when using

---

Box 7.2: Twenty-one possible pitfalls in interviewing

1   Not being thorough enough in gaining consent
2   Not making clear the purpose of the interview
3   Not making clear what the answers will be used for and how that will help the interviewee
4   Interruptions from outside (e.g. telephone, visitors)
5   Competing distractions (e.g. others in the room, children)
6   Stage fright for interviewer
7   Stage fright for interviewee
8   Jumping from one subject to another
9   Lack of logical flow in questions
10   Asking interviewee embarrassing or awkward questions
11   Asking leading or loaded questions
12   Asking imprecise questions
13   Asking questions open to questioning
14   Asking complex questions
15   Teaching (e.g. giving interviewee medical advice)
16   Counselling (e.g. summarising responses too early)
17   Presenting one's own perspective, potentially biasing the interviewee
18   Superficial interviews
19   Ethical issues: what do you do if you receive specific allegations, contradictory information or secret information?
20   Deviating from the main objectives of the interview
21   Translations from the interview's story and reinterpreting it in your own words

---

questionnaires. Table 7.3 gives an indication of categories of questions that can be found in clinical research and clinical practice. It also provides examples and suggestions for improvement.

In protocol-driven, ethically approved research most of the problems with the questions should have been sorted out before the trial is started. However all of the above examples have been seen in research with and without lay involvement. So there is no guarantee that just because a research project has ethical approval to start that it will be free of problems in its questions. Table 7.3 has a variety of uses. It:

• shows you a diversity of types of questions
• indicates that the type of question could predetermine the particular answer given

Table 7.3: Types of questions for questionnaires

Type of question	Example	Suggestions for improvement
Open	From your experience, what key messages would you offer to those planning a phase three double-blind placebo-controlled parallel clinical trial in primary care for the treatment of insomnia?	Check the respondent understands the terminology in the question, get background information about their clinical trial experience, determine the time scale (was it a trial they were involved in some time ago, one they are just finishing being part of, or one they are still heavily involved in?) Think about whom the answer(s) will be relayed to. Pick out a particular trial, and then ask a more specific question about their key messages. Because it is an open question be aware that the respondent may give a lot of answers, or they may give very few answers and that any answer they do give could be vague in the actual detail. More questions should be asked to tease out the respondent's key messages.
Closed	What was the length of time, in minutes, between the patient with myocardial infarction (MI) arriving at the emergency unit and their receiving thrombolytic therapy?	Think about whether the patient could have received the treatment on the way to hospital – e.g. in an ambulance. Try to trace when the MI started, who was called to attend, who attended, who diagnosed the condition, what specific interventions were given (dose etc), and when.
Leading	Your family doctor, who is very good at his work, has done everything possible to help you in this trial, are you happy with your care?	Provide evidence of how good the doctor is (e.g. independent clinical audit reviews, qualifications, trial experience and testimonies), provide evidence of what was done, provide evidence of what could have been done (e.g. outside the trial), provide evidence of the trial protocol and standard operating procedures, and then specifically ask a series of questions relating to the care and satisfaction.
Imprecise	Did you arrive at the hospital quickly after developing chest pains?	Find out when the pains started, where the person was when they started, how they got to the hospital, when they got there, and who they saw on arrival.
Open to interpretation	Did the surgeon tell you what was going to happen after the trial?	Make sure the respondent knows who the surgeon is, find out what information was provided by whom, when and in what form, find out what happened, establish the points in time, then ask a more specific question.

Table 7.3: Continued

Type of question	Example	Suggestions for improvement
Composite	Did you understand and follow the clinical trial protocol completely?	Split the question into separate parts. Did you know what the trial protocol was? Did you understand the trial protocol? Did you follow the protocol completely?
Double negative	Would you not have preferred not to be asked to join the trial?	Disentangle. Would you have preferred not to be asked to join the trial?
Presumptuous	How long have you been having unprotected sex?	Avoid making unnecessary presumptions. Split the question into whether or not they have had unprotected sex, then ask relevant questions about time scales, frequency, type of sex (vaginal, anal) number of partners.

- illustrates the point that one question could lead to a whole series of other questions
- makes you aware of the need to be vigilant as to what questions were or are being asked e.g. in committee, research publications, trial protocols, during patient interaction
- makes you think about what type of question should have been asked
- encourages you to think harder about your own questions before you ask them.

Action research

Over the last 50 years action research has been described and defined in various ways by different people (e.g. Lewin, Corey, and Hopkins to name a few). In 1994 for example, Calhoun suggested that it was 'a fancy way of saying let's study what's happening and decide how to make it a better place'.[9]

Action research is a family of methodologies which jointly pursues action (or change) and research (or understanding) at the same time. It seeks to be a virtuous spiral of action and of research. The spiral involves cycles. As Figure 7.1 shows, each cycle involves reconnaissance, planning, action and reflection. In the later cycles, action research continuously refines the methods, data and interpretation in the light of the evidence and understanding developed in the earlier cycles.

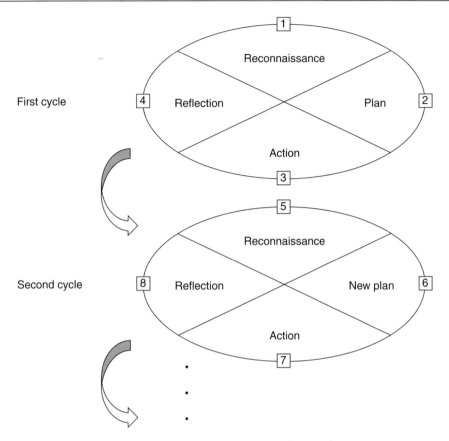

Figure 7.1: An action research spiral.

- **Reconnaissance**: an exploratory stance is adopted, where specification and understanding of the problem is developed.
- **Plan**: plans are made for some form of intervention strategy.
- **Action**: after negotiation and discussion with interested parties, the intervention is carried out.
- **Reflection and revision**: evaluation of the intervention and re-evaluation of the initial problem.

Before, during and after each intervention, observations are made and information is collected and analysed. Action research generally involves a 'look, think, act' process. It is therefore intended to foster a deeper understanding of a given situation, starting with conceptualising and particularising the problem and moving through several actions, reflections, refinements and evaluations. It also makes us think about the contexts we are working in, how they affect our judgements and our interpretations upon which those judgements are based. The spiral process repeats itself until the desired improvements to practice are achieved.

Action research is:

- an *emergent* process that takes shape as understanding increases
- an *iterative* process that converges towards a better understanding of practice and change
- *pragmatic* in terms of action and of research
- *participative* (among other reasons, change is usually easier to achieve when those affected by the change are involved in each cycle)
- *reflective*
- *'evidence-based'* (the research and action are both driven by the evidence from the literature and at hand)
- often a blend of *qualitative* and *quantitative* research and action.

Action research has the potential to generate genuine and sustained improvements in lay involvement in research and professional practice. Action research can offer your team with lay involvement:

- greater feelings of ownership of action and of analysis
- pragmatic insight into real-life issues, ambitions, constraints and solutions
- new opportunities to reflect on and assess work
- scope and structure to explore and test new ideas, methods and materials
- possibilities to assess how effective the new approaches were in context
- positive and constructive opportunities to share feedback with friends and colleagues
- a basis for formulating and acting on the evidence and analysis.

Furthermore, action research is useful for lay involvement strategies because it provides opportunities to find answers to researchers' questions and it can help provide answers to questions being posed by those affected or involved in the issues under study. Working collaboratively can benefit everyone involved and beyond:

- such research requires that parties share information and resources
- refined, reflective and shared goals are considered possible
- it dilutes feelings of powerlessness particularly amongst the otherwise research inactive fraternity, and those solely and rudely confined to 'consumer or user status'
- it promotes co-operation
- it facilitates a more credible and cohesive programme of research, results and implementation

- it offers opportunities for fruitful and subsequent lines of research and enquiry
- it offers scope to depersonalise the data, and at the same time raise the demand for more robust methods and analysis.

In healthcare, action research has been used in:

- lay involvement in research
- enhancing patient information leaflets
- reviving recruitment into research programmes
- restoring asthmatics' compliance with their medication regimen
- adapting clinical research management programmes
- transforming cancer patients' care paths
- reducing medication errors
- enhancing pastoral and moral support services for families in a children's hospital
- developing physiotherapy services for the elderly and newly disabled
- improving training and induction programmes for new members of ethics committees
- managing patient and practitioner change from one medicine to another
- developing nurse-led disease-management clinics
- refining dispensing pharmacists' interaction and involvement with patients, nurses and doctors in repeat prescribing programmes.

Action research has also been used in areas such as law and order, and social care and is, currently, a popular approach in the field of education.

References

1   Earl-Slater A (2002) *The Handbook of Clinical Trials and Other Research.* Radcliffe Medical Press, Oxford.

2   Ely JW, Dawson JD, Young PR *et al.* (1999) Malpractice claims against family physicians: are the best doctors sued more? *J Fam Pract.* **48**: 23–30.

3   Glasgow RE, Showstack J, Katz PP *et al.* (1999) The relationship between hospital volume and outcomes of hepatic resection for hepatocellular carcinoma. *Arch Surg.* **134**: 30–5.

4   Reid S, Wessely S, Crayford T and Hotopf M (2001) Medially unexplained symptoms in frequent attenders of secondary health care: retrospective cohort study. *BMJ.* **322**: 767.

5   Doll R, Peto R, Boreham J and Sutherland J (2000) Smoking and dementia in male British doctors: a prospective study. *BMJ.* **320**: 1097–102.

6 Evans J, Heron J, Francomb H *et al.* (2001) Cohort study of depressed mood during pregnancy and after childbirth. *BMJ.* **323**: 257–60.

7 Freemantle N, Eccles M, Wood J *et al.* (1999) A randomised trial of evidence-based outreach (EBOR) rationale and design. *Control Clin Trials.* **20**: 479–92.

8 Montgomery AA, Fahey T, Peters TJ *et al.* (2000) Evaluation of computer-based clinical support systems and risk chart. *BMJ.* **320**: 686–90.

9 Earl-Slater A (2002) The superiority of action research. *Br J Clin Gov.* **7**: 132–5.

Further reading

- Bowling A (1997) *Research Methods in Health: investigating health and health services.* Open University Press, Buckingham.
- Stringer ET (1996) *Action Research: a handbook for practitioners.* Sage Publications, London.

Chapter 8

Questions to ask before getting involved in research

Before you and your research team get involved in a particular research study there are various questions that you must ask. If you are inviting a lay person to become involved in your research team be prepared to answer the following questions that they and other members of the team may have (*see* Box 8.1).

Many of the questions in Box 8.1 can be used by a variety of people. For example the questions can be used by:

- healthcare professionals to quiz the principal investigator
- healthcare professionals to quiz the study sponsor (and vice versa)
- one healthcare professional to another
- a healthcare manager to doctors thinking of taking part in the trial in their organisation
- a healthcare manager to a study sponsor
- prospective lay members to anyone in the research team, especially the lead researcher, host organisation and study sponsor
- the ethics review committee to the principal investigator
- patients to the doctor
- patients to the principal investigator.

Although Box 8.1 is already long and interesting, it is not comprehensive. There will be other questions that you yourself can think of asking.

From experience, you may have been tempted to skip through Box 8.1. If you have skipped through it, then you have not really done yourself or your research team any favours, personally or professionally.

The 'fate of clinical trials research' pyramid

Figure 8.1 presents the 'fate of clinical trials research' pyramid. This pyramid has been the starting point of many questions that can and should be asked about a research project. So if you are planning a project

Box 8.1: Questions to ask before getting involved in a clinical trial

1   What is the primary research question?
2   Why is the research being done?
3   What do the researchers want to accomplish?
4   What is already known about the intervention(s)?
5   What is already known about the disease?
6   What are the study entry and exclusion criteria?
7   What evidence exists to support the entry and exclusion criteria?
8   What type of study is it?
9   What evidence supports that type of study?
10 What is the system of recruitment?
11 What is the system of allocation to arms in the study, if any?
12 What will be done during the trial and for how long?
13 What risks are involved in the study?
14 What benefits can be expected from the study?
15 What other treatments are available?
16 If a patient refuses to enter will they still get access to the product?
17 How do the possible risks and benefits of the trial compare to current practice?
18 What data will be collected?
19 How will data be collected?
20 Who will analyse the data?
21 What will be done with the data after the study has finished?
22 What is the plan for disseminating the study results?
23 Will I see a summary of the results before they are published?
24 Where will the results of the trial be published?
25 Where is the study site?
26 How often do I have to attend?
27 What do I have to do when I am there?
28 Will I receive any payment?
29 What are my responsibilities during the study?
30 What happens if things get worse during the study?
31 Can I talk to anyone about the study?
32 Can anyone else find out I am in the study?
33 What happens to the patients after the study has finished?
34 What happens if I want to leave the study early?
35 What happens if not enough patients are recruited?
36 What happens if recruitment is slower than expected?
37 What happens to the patients if the study is stopped early?

38   Who is sponsoring the study?
39   Why are they sponsoring the study?
40   Who has reviewed the study?
41   Who has approved the study?
42   Does the trial meet ethical, regulatory and legal requirements?
43   Who is the principal investigator?
44   What skills and experience do the research team actually have?
45   Can I have a copy of the study protocol?
46   Is anyone in the research team soliciting or receiving commission or rewards (monetary or otherwise) for getting me involved in this research?

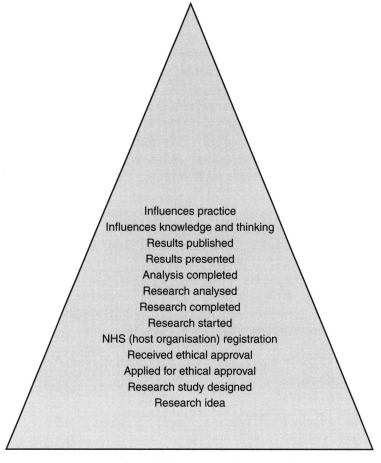

Figure 8.1: The 'fate of clinical trials research' pyramid.

use the pyramid as part of your business framework to outline time scales, resources, barriers and opportunities to taking the work forward. Also use it as a pictorial device to help establish and answer questions that others may ask about your research.

The 'fate of research' pyramid runs up from the base initial idea for the study, up to its highest point, influencing clinical practice. There are various stages between these points as highlighted in the pyramid.

Reading from the base up, the pyramid suggests that there are many more research study ideas than there are studies designed. Moving further up the pyramid you will see that not all studies that are designed get ethical approval. This is not necessarily bad news as failure to get research approval can signal legitimate concerns with the research idea, plan or its methods. It would be quite unethical to approve a faulty or defective research application. There is however no comprehensive database of research application failures, the reasons for failure, and therefore no memory or databank from which other researchers, the NHS or research approval committees can learn. Nor is there any robust and comprehensive database of research application successes. The evolving National Research Register (*see* Appendix 1) is a good start but you will find that it is not comprehensive and it does not give any indication of what actually happened to the research.

For various reasons, not all research that is started is completed, and not all studies that are completed are analysed, presented or published.

While the highest point in the pyramid is taken by studies that influence practice, remember that many things, in a complex way, affect clinical practice. Interpretation of results from clinical studies is just one of the possible influences.

You should not enter into a research study lightly, as they are serious scientific experiments. Equally you should never be afraid to ask questions about the study. This will show you are taking the idea of the study seriously.

Make your own questions count. The most important thing is that you ask questions and feel comfortable about the answers. It is usually a very good idea to get the answers in writing from the appropriate authority.

If you are unhappy or unclear about any of the answers, ask again, and if you are still not sure, discuss this with your colleagues and friends. If you are in any serious doubt, stay out of that study. Even if you do go into a study, you are not locked inextricably into it – if for any reason you wish to leave, best practice suggests you talk to the lead researcher and if you still want to leave, leave.

Further reading

- Altman DG (1994) The scandal of poor medical research. *BMJ*. **308**: 283–4.
- Easterbrook PJ and Mathews DR (1992) Fate of research studies. *J R Soc Med*. **85**: 71–6.
- Earl-Slater A (2002) *The Handbook of Clinical Trials and Other Research*. Radcliffe Medical Press, Oxford.
- Earl-Slater A (2001) The EU Clinical Trials Directive. *J R Soc Med*. **94**: 557–8.
- Earl-Slater A (2002) The superiority of action research. *Br J Clin Gov*. **7**: 132–5.
- Good CS (ed) (1976) *The Principles and Practice of Clinical Trials*. Churchill Livingston, London.
- Prescott RJ, Counsell CE, Gillespie WJ *et al*. (1999) Factors that limit quality, number and progress of randomised controlled trials. *Health Technol Assess*. **3**(20).
- The Wellcome Trust and London Regional Office of the NHS Executive (2001) *Putting NHS research on the Map: an analysis of scientific publications in England: 1990–1997*. The Wellcome Trust and The London Regional Office of the NHS Executive, London, May 2001 (available at www.wellcome.ac.uk or by email to marketing@wellcome.ac.uk).
- Thomas P (2000) The research needs of primary care: trials must be relevant to patients. *BMJ*. **321**: 2–3.
- Tognini G, Alli C, Avanzini F *et al*. (1991) Randomised clinical trials in general practice: lessons from a failure. *BMJ*. **303**: 969–71.
- Ward E, King M, Lloyd M *et al*. (1999) Conducting randomised trials in general practice: methodological and practical issues. *Br J Gen Pract*. **49**: 919–22.
- Wilson S, Delaney BC, Roalfe A *et al*. (2000) Randomised controlled trials in primary care: case study. *BMJ*. **321**: 24–7.
- Wise P and Drury M (1996) Pharmaceutical trials in general practice: the first 100 protocols. An audit by the clinical research ethics committee of the Royal College of General Practitioners. *BMJ*. **313**: 1245–8.

Chapter 9

Regulation of patient data: Caldicott Guardians

In research as in clinical practice, serious attention has to be paid to data handling. As you know there is of course the Data Protection Act, which everyone in the research team should be conversant with (*see* Chapter 10). Adding to that framework of law is the 'Caldicott Guardians'. The Caldicott Guardians first made their appearance throughout the NHS from April 1999. You and your research team need to know that their principal duty is to safeguard and protect the handling of confidential patient information as it passes between and out of NHS organisations.

The Caldicott Committee was set up in response to a threatened British Medical Association boycott of the NHS 'net' because of the vulnerability of patient data flowing from clinical to administrative settings. Led by Dame Fiona Caldicott, principal of Somerville College, Oxford, and past president of the Royal College of Psychiatrists, the Caldicott Committee report appeared in 1997.[1]

The introduction of 'local guardians of patient confidentiality' was a key recommendation of the Caldicott report, and an NHS Executive circular ordered NHS units to have them appointed by 1 April 1999.[2] Each health authority, NHS trust, and primary care group appointed the individuals in what has become a network of Caldicott Guardians. The NHS circular said that ideally the guardians should be board members and senior health professionals, with some responsibility for clinical governance within the organisation. According to the NHS Executive circular their work should not be delegated: '*It is intended that Caldicott Guardians will be central to the development of a new framework for handling patient information in the NHS*'.[2]

In support of the Caldicott Guardians, NHS boards developed protocols for:

- the disclosure of patient information to other organisations
- access to data
- reviewing the uses of patient data
- improving database design, staff training, and compliance.

The Caldicott report offered six principles of good practice for the health service when handling patient-identifiable information (*see* Box 9.1). These are very important, and everyone in your research team should be aware of and adhere to them.

Caldicott Guardians should have the authority to exercise the necessary influence on local policy and strategic planning in the NHS. Candidates might include directors of public health and clinical or nursing directors of trusts. Each primary care group and trust should have its Caldicott Guardian, and each practice should nominate a liaison point for confidentiality issues. Preserving patient confidentiality is

---

Box 9.1: Caldicott principles of good practice

- **Principle 1 Justify the purpose(s):**
  - every proposed use or transfer of patient-identifiable information within or from an organisation should be clearly defined and scrutinised, with continuing uses regularly reviewed by an appropriate guardian.
- **Principle 2 Do not use patient-identifiable information unless it is absolutely necessary:**
  - patient-identifiable information items should not be used unless there is no alternative.
- **Principle 3 Use the minimum necessary patient-identifiable information:**
  - where use of patient-identifiable information is considered to be essential, each individual item of information should be justified with the aim of reducing identifiability.
- **Principle 4 Access to patient-identifiable information should be on a strict need-to-know basis:**
  - only those individuals who need access to patient-identifiable information should have access to it, and they should only have access to the information items that they need to see.
- **Principle 5 Everyone should be aware of their responsibilities**
  - action should be taken to ensure that those handling patient-identifiable information – both clinical and non-clinical staff – are aware of their responsibilities and obligations to respect patient confidentiality.
- **Principle 6 Understand and comply with the law**
  - every use of patient-identifiable information must be lawful. Someone in each organisation should be responsible for ensuring that the organisation complies with legal requirements.

---

considered a cornerstone of the NHS information strategy. The then Junior Health Minister Baroness Hayman said that the Caldicott Guardians would have a vital role to play as the NHS learns to harness the enormous potential of information technology. Dr Ian Bogle, as chairman of council of the BMA, welcomed the initiative. In 1999 Dr Bogle is reported to have said that the process had a long way to go but that the setting up of a system of guardians was a vital first step. Dr Sandy Macara, then chairman of the British Medical Association reportedly said 'there is still much to be done, but we can all now see where the start line is'. However Dr Fleur Fisher of the Campaign for Medical Privacy is reported as saying 'we still have databases built in an unacceptable and unethical way'.

It is clear that the six principles in Box 9.1 can be used in any research study whether or not there is lay involvement. Again I stress that these six principles should be made clear to everyone in your research team.

The health service circular on Caldicott Guardians is available from the Department of Health: http://www.open.gov.uk/doh/coinh.htm.

References

1 Caldicott Committee (1997) *Report on the Review of Patient Identifiable Information.* Department of Health, London.
2 NHS Executive (1999) *Protecting and Using Patient Information: a manual for Caldicott Guardians.* NHS Executive, London.

Further reading

* Anderson R (2001) Undermining data privacy in health information. *BMJ.* **322**: 442–3.
* Carnall D (1997) Report urges widespread reform of handling NHS data. *BMJ.* **315**: 1559.
* Earl-Slater A (2002) *The Handbook of Clinical Trials and Other Research.* Radcliffe Medical Press, Oxford.
* Mandl KD, Szolovits P, Kohane IS *et al.* (2001) Public standards and patients' control: how to keep electronic medical records accessible but private. *BMJ.* **322**: 283–7.
* Strobl J, Cave E and Walley T (2000) Data protection legislation: interpretation and barriers to research. *BMJ.* **321**: 890–2.
* Warden J (1999) Guardians to protect patient data. *BMJ.* **318**: 284.
* Willison DJ, Keshavjee K, Nair K *et al.* (2003) Patients' consent preferences for research uses of information in electronic medical records: interview and survey data. *BMJ.* **326**: 373–6.

Chapter 10

Research ethics committees

If the research you are getting involved in has not received and will not seek research ethics committee approval be very wary of joining that research team. Best practice suggests that an independent research ethics committee should review the research proposal. In the healthcare sector you should always seek ethics committee approval – some funders make it mandatory and most healthcare organisations compel you to do so. It is in your own best interests as a professional and a researcher to have your research reviewed by an ethics committee.

The purpose of this chapter is to provide an outline of two types of committees – local research ethics committees and multicentre research ethics committees. As part of the EU there is a directive covering clinical research of medicinal products and you must keep up to date with developments in that area.

Guidance was issued by the Department of Health during 1991 requiring each of the then district health authorities to establish by February 1992 a local research ethics committee (LREC). LRECs are neither a management arm of the health authority nor a sub-committee of any other committee.

The general purpose of an LREC is:

- to maintain ethical standards of practice in research, and to ensure that guidelines issued by relevant bodies are adhered to
- to protect subjects of research from harm
- to preserve the subject's rights
- to provide reassurance to the public that these aims are being met.

LRECs have been consulted on the ethical issues of a proposed research project where it involves:

- NHS patients, including those under contracts with private sector providers
- foetal material and in vitro fertilisation (IVF) involving NHS patients
- the recently dead, in NHS premises
- access to the records of past or present NHS patients
- use of, or potential access to, NHS premises or facilities.

Audits and clinical governance investigations are two types of analysis that have not usually been sent to LRECs for consideration. This does not mean that these types of analysis could not be improved by independent ratification by such a committee.

From experience, if there is any doubt about the suitability of a study for ethical review then the researcher should actively seek the advice of the chairman of the committee well in advance of commencing the study.

Any investigator who bypasses or ignores the recommendations of a properly authorised ethics committee does in fact create a potentially serious situation. They create for themselves a situation that could make them vulnerable to professional disciplinary or even legal proceedings. In addition to this, if their study is flawed they will be wasting patients', administrators' and their colleagues' time. Developments in research governance in the NHS mean that NHS organisations must be aware of what research is being undertaken in their organisation.

LRECs submit an annual report to the health authority. This includes details such as the number of meetings held and a list of the proposals considered (including whether they were approved, approved after amendment, rejected or withdrawn). Copies of the report are sent to other NHS parties and are made available for public inspection.

A typical LREC may have the following members: two lay persons (one acting as chairman or vice-chairman); two general practitioners; one from the nursing profession; three medical practitioners from the local NHS hospital(s), a medical practitioner from the community (non-general practice) and a pharmacist. The membership should be representative of both sexes and cover a wide experience. Members do not, and should not, act in a representative capacity. Appointments are usually for an initial period of three years. Some LRECs have excellent induction programmes for new members.

While the members should cover a wide experience, LRECs may seek the advice of specialist referees or co-opt members to the committee so as to cover any aspect (e.g. professional, scientific or ethical) of a research proposal that lies beyond the expertise of the existing members. Investigators are asked to attend the meeting where their application is being discussed. This is especially true where there is a complicated or controversial proposal.

More details on LRECs can be found on the Central Office for Research Ethics Committees website (COREC) at http://www.corec.org.uk.

Multicentre research ethics committee

A new system for obtaining ethical approval for multicentre research was announced in the 1997 Health Service Guidelines document.[1] In order to facilitate the process of ethical review of multicentre research, multicentre research ethics committees (MRECs) were established in 1997 to complement the work of existing LRECs.

The MREC system is an attempt to solve various problems of multilocation research. These include:

- a diversity of local ethical requirements and systems
- multiplicity of applications
- delayed time to receive decisions
- variations in decisions
- duplication of effort
- lack of co-ordination.

The MREC system would, it was hoped, facilitate useful research, raise the standards, and dilute the problems outlined above.

In addition then, the general purpose of an MREC is:

- to maintain ethical standards of practice in research, and to ensure that guidelines issued by relevant bodies are adhered to
- to protect subjects of research from harm
- to preserve the subject's rights
- to provide reassurance to the public that these aims are being met.

For the new system, multicentre research is defined as that which is carried out within five or more LRECs' geographical boundaries. All such research must be considered by an MREC.

The MREC application should be made by a single named 'principal researcher', to the NHS region within which they are based. Interestingly, the decision of the MREC will then apply to all regions in England. Reciprocal arrangements are in place with similar committees established in Scotland, Wales and Northern Ireland.

Once MREC approval has been obtained, the principal researcher will receive a letter of approval which must be sent to any local researchers who are to be involved. The local researchers must then submit the application, together with the MREC approval, to the LREC, for consideration of issues that may affect local acceptability. LRECs will not consider applications for multicentre research without the MREC approval letter.

The MRECs in each region are given the responsibility of reviewing research proposals taking place within the boundaries of five or more

LRECs. The study need not involve a clinical trial: for example it could involve a plan for database research, patient interviews or pharmacy practice observation. Interestingly, approval by one MREC for the research would have national acceptance. However even with such approval there is no compulsion to do the trial on a national scale.

The MRECs have been established in accordance with the advice given in two NHS publications[1,2] and in the context of the guidance given in documents MEL (1997) 8, HSG (91) 5 and circular 1992 (GEN) 93. As of February 1998, the standing orders for MRECs in the UK NHS are as follows:

The committee will be responsible for considering multicentre research where the principal researcher is based in the relevant area and the research is to be conducted within five or more LRECs' geographical boundaries.

Membership

The chairman and vice-chairman are appointed by the Chief Medical Officer and one of these appointments is to be lay. They will serve initially for two years and will be reappointed in such a way as to ensure continuity of experience. Members will serve for a period of three to five years, renewable for one term. The composition of the MREC is set out in Table 10.1.

The chairman has the authority, in consultation with the Department of Health and the membership, to approach any member whose conduct is felt to be detrimental to the cohesion and work of the committee and to discuss this matter for the benefit of the whole committee. Ultimately, if this cannot be resolved the member can be asked to resign.

Attendance at meetings

Members should not have deputies. If a member fails to attend three consecutive meetings or less than 50% of the meetings taking place in the year he/she will be deemed to have resigned.

Legal liability

The Department of Health will indemnify MREC members in respect of any loss which they may incur resulting from any claim made against them arising out of the exercise of their function as a member of the MREC, including their legal costs and any compensation and expenses for which they may be found to be liable, provided that the member notifies the department of any such claim and assists it in all reasonable ways.

Declaration of interest

If a member of the committee has a financial or personal interest in a project or with a project sponsor, he/she must inform the chairman who will decide whether the interest disqualifies the member from the discussion.

Confidentiality

Members will keep confidential all paperwork and discussions connected with the work of the MREC.

Accountability

The MREC will be accountable to the Secretary of State – in practice this function has been delegated to the Chief Medical Officer. The main formal mechanism for achieving accountability will be an annual report.

Number and frequency of meetings

The MREC will meet as often as is reasonable and consistent with its workload. This will be initially on a monthly basis.

Agenda papers

Agenda papers will be sent to members, wherever possible, at least two weeks before the meeting at which they will be discussed.

Dates of meetings

Dates of all meetings will be published for the year ahead to enable researchers to target meeting dates. Researchers should send applications to the MREC administrator three weeks before the meeting being targeted.

Attendance at meetings by researchers

Applicants may be asked to attend the MREC meeting at which their project is discussed.

Decisions of the committee

The decisions of the committee will be reached by full discussion of all the ethical issues. Wherever possible a consensus will be reached. All decisions will be notified to the researcher in writing within 10 working days of the meeting at which the project is discussed. Reasons for approval or rejection will always be given. Any significant minority view will be noted in the minutes and the comments may be forwarded to the researcher anonymously if it is thought to be helpful.

The following decisions on an application may be taken:

1 **Approve** – the application is granted ethical approval without amendment.
2 **Approve subject to amendment** – the application is granted ethical approval subject to relatively minor amendments and authority is delegated to the chairman to confirm that the response received from the principal researcher conforms with the committee's requirements.
3 **Defer** – consideration of the application is deferred to a future meeting pending receipt of substantial amendments, clarification or further information.
4 **Reject** – the application is refused ethical approval as it is intrinsically unethical and not capable of easy amendment.
5 **Transfer** – the application is not appropriate for the particular MREC and will be transferred to a more appropriate one.

General conditions of approval

The MREC will offer ethical approval subject to the following general conditions:

- there is no divergence from the original protocol without first contacting the committee
- regular updates of the progress of the research and a report of the outcome of the trial are received

- the project is started within three years of the date approval is given; extensions can be applied for
- adverse events are notified to the MREC, relevant LRECs and the sponsor, using the procedure set out in the MREC guidelines.

MREC cross-referrals

A heavily loaded MREC may, by agreement between the secretariats, pass work to another MREC. Proposals may also be passed to another committee where an MREC has expertise in a specialised area. No MREC can hear appeals against another MREC or LREC. Any differences between a researcher and MREC must be resolved between themselves. It will be possible to seek referral to another MREC if an outcome cannot be resolved, providing there is agreement with the initial MREC and researcher. The advice of the second MREC will be final.

Chairman's action

Chairman's action will never be used to decide an initial proposal. It is appropriate for confirming minor amendments in applications approved subject to amendment where the principal researcher has fulfilled the requirements. It is also appropriate for determining whether amendments to applications already approved are sufficiently substantive to require consideration by the full committee or whether they are sufficiently minor to be approved by chairman's action. Decisions made under chairman's action should be reported to the next meeting of the committee.

Quorum

A quorum will consist of half of the members, providing it includes either the chairman or vice-chairman, at least two lay members and two medically qualified members. The administrator should ensure each meeting will be quorate prior to the meeting.

Minutes of meetings

Minutes will be taken of all committee meetings. These will be confidential but may be sent to the Chief Medical Officer, Chief Scientist and LREC chairmen on request.

Retention of applications

The administrator of the MREC will retain copies of all applications received by the committee for a period of three years beyond the conclusion of the research.

Annual report

An annual report will be sent to the Secretary of State or his representative. Copies of the annual report will also be available to LREC chairmen and the Department of Health. The annual report will be available for public inspection.

Reviewing approved research

The MREC will expect to be advised of any adverse results, failure to complete research or any other information that may be considered of interest to the MREC in the conduct of its work. In addition the MREC requires an annual progress report and a final report on completion of the project. Pro forma are provided in the guidelines for this purpose. The researcher is also required to advise the MREC if the research is withdrawn or if difficulties are experienced in recruiting research subjects.

Application fee

An application fee of £1000 per application will be charged for research sponsored by commercial companies.

Figure 10.1 provides an illustration of a flowchart for a MREC system.

Table 10.1 sets out the composition for the MRECs. In practice, variations of composition within agreed parameters are permissible.

In September 1998 the NHS Executive issued points of guidance to LRECs stating that:

- a standing sub-committee of the LREC should be established to consider applications approved by MRECs (quorum shall be two members)
- a meeting of this LREC executive sub-committee should be called within two weeks of receipt of an application approved by a MREC

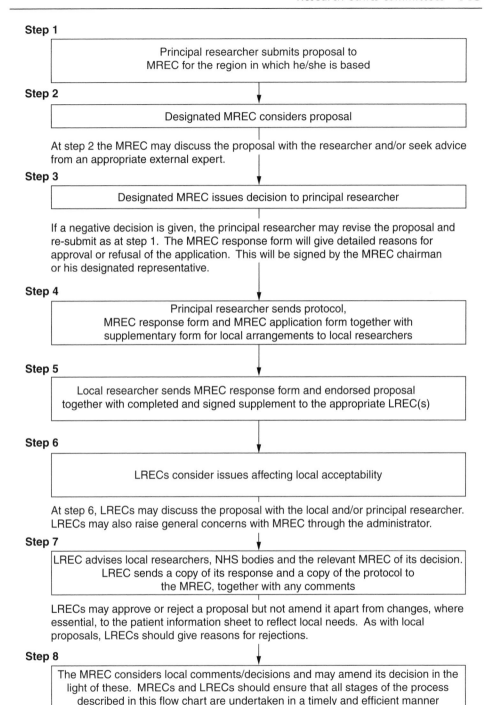

Step 1

> Principal researcher submits proposal to
> MREC for the region in which he/she is based

Step 2

> Designated MREC considers proposal

At step 2 the MREC may discuss the proposal with the researcher and/or seek advice from an appropriate external expert.

Step 3

> Designated MREC issues decision to principal researcher

If a negative decision is given, the principal researcher may revise the proposal and re-submit as at step 1. The MREC response form will give detailed reasons for approval or refusal of the application. This will be signed by the MREC chairman or his designated representative.

Step 4

> Principal researcher sends protocol,
> MREC response form and MREC application form together with
> supplementary form for local arrangements to local researchers

Step 5

> Local researcher sends MREC response form and endorsed proposal
> together with completed and signed supplement to the appropriate LREC(s)

Step 6

> LRECs consider issues affecting local acceptability

At step 6, LRECs may discuss the proposal with the local and/or principal researcher. LRECs may also raise general concerns with MREC through the administrator.

Step 7

> LREC advises local researchers, NHS bodies and the relevant MREC of its decision.
> LREC sends a copy of its response and a copy of the protocol to
> the MREC, together with any comments

LRECs may approve or reject a proposal but not amend it apart from changes, where essential, to the patient information sheet to reflect local needs. As with local proposals, LRECs should give reasons for rejections.

Step 8

> The MREC considers local comments/decisions and may amend its decision in the
> light of these. MRECs and LRECs should ensure that all stages of the process
> described in this flow chart are undertaken in a timely and efficient manner

Figure 10.1: A multicentre research ethics system flowchart
(simplifed example).

Table 10.1: MREC membership

Description	Maximum number	Minimum number
General practitioner	2	1
Nurse/midwife	2	1
Professional allied to medicine	1	1
Clinical pharmacologist/pharmacist	2	1
Hospital consultant	4	3
Public health physician/epidemiologist	1	1
Lay person*	6	4
Total:	18	12

* A person who is not and never has been (i) a doctor, dentist, ophthalmic medical practitioner, optician or pharmacist; (ii) a registered dispensing optician; (iii) a registered nurse, registered midwife or registered health visitor; (iv) an officer of, or someone otherwise employed by any health board, health authority, local health council or community health council.

- the decision of the LREC executive sub-committee should be communicated to the researcher within five working days. This does not require ratification by the full committee, and if approval is granted, the research work may commence
- rejection of the application by the LREC executive sub-committee can only be for local reasons (see below) and must be accompanied by a full explanation for this decision.

Reasons for LREC rejection could be based on:

- the suitability of the local researcher
- the suitability of the site
- the suitability of the subjects
- requiring that the patient information sheets and consent forms are to carry local information as required or to be produced in a locally appropriate language. No other changes to the information sheets or consent forms can be made.

Exactly what is meant by the term 'suitability' remains unclear. Some studies are reported to have been deemed 'unsuitable' by one LREC but not by another LREC. This divergence in opinion could be for legitimate reasons: further research is required.

One development for MRECs is to use a standard progress report form (see Box 10.1). Such a form is reproduced here as an illustration of what information the MREC would get if these forms were sent out, completed, returned and analysed.

Information from these forms would not only help the trialists provide an update of the status of the trial, but would provide the

Box 10.1: A MREC research progress report

1   Name and address of principal researcher
2   Short title of study
3   Research ethics committee reference number
4   Date of research ethics committee approval
5   Has the study started?   Yes   No
    If no, please give reasons
6   Number of local research sites recruited   Proposed   Actual
7   Number of subjects/patients recruited into study   Proposed   Actual
8   Number of subjects/patients completing study   Proposed   Actual
9   Number of withdrawals because of:
    (i)   lack of efficacy
    (ii) adverse events
    (iii) self-withdrawal
    (iv) non-compliance
10 Have there been any serious difficulties in
    recruiting subjects to the study?   Yes   No
    If yes, please give details
11 Have there been any untoward events?   Yes   No
    (before you answer this, please refer to our definition in the enclosed booklet
    Information for Researchers)
    If Yes, have these been notified to the committee?   Yes   No
12 If untoward events have not been notified to the committee, please state why
    as notification is a condition of research ethics committee approval
13 Have there been any amendments to the study?   Yes   No
    If yes, have these been notified to the committee?   Yes   No
    If amendments have not been notified to the committee, please state why as
    you know that notification is a condition of the committee's approval
14 Has the study finished?   Yes   No
    If yes, please answer questions (15 and 16) below
    If no, what is the expected completion date?
15 If the study will not now be completed, please give reason(s)
16 Results – please include details of outcomes and conclusions (attach a
    separate page if necessary).
    How the findings have been disseminated
    Used for licensing/regulatory purposes   Yes   No
    Presentations   Yes   No
    Publications: planned   Yes   No
                       in press   Yes   No
                       published   Yes   No
    Please give details below and send copies of publications and presentations
    as soon as they are available
17 Signature of principal investigator
18 Print principal investigator's name
19 Signature(s) of the chief executive(s) of the organisation(s) where the research
    takes place
20 Date of submission of progress report to the ethics committee

approving committee with valuable insight into the progress of work they have recommended. More generally that information could be used to help share real lessons and insight into the fate of research to host institutions, non-trial doctors, trial sponsors generally, and of course patients and their advocates.

At the time of writing the MREC system in the UK is very much part of a larger emerging system of ratifying trial applications. As indicated above there is still some work to do in terms of actually monitoring the approved trials, monitoring the system of approving trials, making the ethics committees' decisions more transparent, and in encouraging the results of trials ratified by NHS ethics committees using NHS patients to be better disseminated publicly.

The clinical research ethics committee system in the UK is undergoing another period of reflection, revision and reform. It is doing this under the guise of improvements to research governance in the NHS and in light of the EU directive on clinical trials of medicinal products for humans. Exactly what new system emerges, why, and how well it does, remains to be seen.

Finally, everyone actively involved in the research team needs to be aware of the work and procedures of the research ethics committees.

References

1 NHS Executive (1997) *Ethics Committee Review of Multi-Centre Research: establishment of multi-centre research ethics committees.* NHS Executive Health Service Guidelines, HSG(97)23, NHS Executive, Leeds.

2 MREC Central Office (2000) *Revised MREC Paperwork.* NHS Executive, South Thames, London.

Further reading

- Ah-See KW, MacKenzie J, Thakker NS *et al.* (1998) Local research ethics committee approval for a national study in Scotland. *J R Coll Surg Edinb.* **43**: 303–5.
- Alberti KGMM (1995) Local research ethics committees. *BMJ.* **311**: 639–41.
- Alberti KGMM (2000) Multicentre research ethics committees: has the cure been worse than the disease? *BMJ.* **320**: 1157–8.
- Busby A and Dolk H (1998) Local research ethics committees' approval in a national population study. *J Roy Coll Physicians Lond.* **32**: 142–5.

- Earl-Slater A (2001) The EU clinical trials directive. *J Roy Soc Med.* **94**: 557–8.
- Earl-Slater A (2002) *The Handbook of Clinical Trials and Other Research.* Radcliffe Medical Press, Oxford.
- Earl-Slater A (2002) Research governance and the fate of research. *Br J Clin Gov.* **7**: 57–62.
- Lux AL, Edwards SW and Osborne JP (2000) Responses of local research ethics committees to a study with approval from a multicentre research ethics committee. *BMJ.* **320**: 1182–3.
- NHS Executive (1998) *Guidance Points to Local Research Ethics Committees.* NHS Executive, Leeds.
- Tulley J, Ninis N, Booy R *et al.* (2000) The new system of review by multicentre research ethics committees: prospective study. *BMJ.* **320**: 1179–82.
- While AE (1995) Ethics committees: impediments to research or guardians of ethical standards? *BMJ.* **311**: 661.

Chapter 11

Human rights and ethics: guidelines and contacts

As yet there is no hard evidence to suggest how ethics committees view lay people's involvement in research. Do they require lay involvement in research applications submitted to them? Do they make it harder or easier for the research to get approval if there is lay involvement? Have any of them made contact with lay people in research in order to indicate how the ethics committees operate and what is required under their current set of standards and procedures? Or is it being left to the lead researchers to furnish the information to lay people (and if so how do the leads know what the ethics committee thinks about lay people's involvement in research?). What training and information are provided to lay people in terms of understanding the practicalities of ethics committees? These questions are becoming increasingly important because of the push for more lay people to become involved in research.

This chapter provides additional information on human rights and data protection. If lay people are to become more involved in research, some awareness of these issues seems necessary. But it is not just lay people that need this information: everyone in the research team needs to be up to the same high level of knowledge and understanding. This indicates to me that at an early stage of any research, a continuing professional development opportunity is offered to the team. Finally, it is strongly advised that you dig into each of the areas to get a clearer and more complete understanding of the topics.

Information about ethics committees, structures and procedures is available from:

- **Central Office For Research Ethics Committees**. On behalf of the Department of Health in England, the Central Office for Research Ethics Committees (COREC) primarily works to co-ordinate the development of operational systems for research ethics committees (RECs) in the National Health Service. COREC's website includes material on research governance, application forms, guidance notes, meeting dates for MRECs, contact information for MRECs and LRECs, and links to other sites of interest, http://www.corec.org.uk.

- **The Association of Research Ethics Committees (AREC)**. AREC is an independent, self-governing body of research ethics committees' members and administrators (local and multicentre). It offers meetings, training and advice for its members, and representation of its members' views in the light of changes to research governance, http://www.arec.org.uk.
- **World Health Organization Operational Guidelines for Ethics Committees that Review Biomedical Research (2000)**. http://who.int/tdr/publications/.

Rights and obligations in research information can be found at:

- **The World Medical Association (WMA) – Declaration Of Helsinki**. Adopted by the 18th WMA General Assembly, Helsinki, Finland, June 1964, amended various times, most recently at the 52nd WMA General Assembly, Edinburgh, Scotland, October 2000, http://www.wma.net.

Some relevant human rights guidelines and information is available from:

- **The Human Rights Act 1998**. This act gives effect to rights and freedoms guaranteed under the European Convention on Human Rights. The rights and fundamental freedoms set out are detailed in the convention and other articles in various protocols, http://www.hmso.gov.uk/acts.
  - Article 2 Right to life
  - Article 3 Prohibition of torture
  - Article 4 Prohibition of slavery and forced labour
  - Article 5 Right to liberty and security
  - Article 6 Right to a fair trial
  - Article 7 No punishment without law
  - Article 8 Right to respect for private and family life
  - Article 9 Freedom of thought, conscience and religion
  - Article 10 Freedom of expression
  - Article 11 Freedom of assembly and association
  - Article 14 Prohibition of discrimination
- **The Council of Europe Convention for the Protection of Human Rights and Dignity of the Human Being with Regards to the Application of Biology and Medicine – Convention on Human Rights and Biomedicine (ETS164)**. The interest of human beings must come before the interest of science or society. Various principles and prohibitions seek to preserve and protect human dignity, rights and freedoms covering issues such as bioethics, medical research, organ

transplantation and consent, http://conventions.coe.int/Treaty [search for ETS164].

- **Department of Health consultation on the draft additional protocol to the Council of Europe Convention on Human Rights and Biomedicine in Biomedical Research**. The convention is to be supplemented by a range of protocols addressing specific issues, http://www.doh.gov.uk/research.

Data and information legislation can be found at:

- **The Data Protection Act 1998**. This covers the processing of information relating to individuals, including obtaining, holding, use and disclosure of such information. It sets out a number of data protection principles, http://www.dataprotection.gov.uk.
- **The Freedom of Information Act 2000**. This act covers the disclosure of information held by public authorities or by persons providing services for them, http://www.hmso.gov.uk/acts/acts2000.
- **Department of Health – Using Confidential Patient Information in the Modern NHS. Caldicott Report and related guidance**. This can be found at http://www.doh.gov.uk. A short introduction is provided in Chapter 9.

Various research councils provide information and guidance on standards and ethics, for example try:

- **The General Medical Council – Standards of Practice**. Information at this link is primarily related to clinical medical practice and research but there are important and useful documents, accessed through the drop down menu 'more about standards of practice . . .', on 'medical research guidance'; 'confidentiality'; and 'consent', http://www.gmc-uk.org/standards.
- **The Medical Research Council**. Although the focus is primarily medical, this site has a number of relevant documents which can be accessed through the link to 'ethics guides' on the welcome page. The guidance on personal information in medical research is one of the most relevant, http://www.mrc.ac.uk.
- **Nuffield Council on Bioethics**. The Nuffield Council on Bioethics is an independent body established in 1991. Its terms of reference require it to consider ethical issues raised by new developments in medicine and biology. It has published a number of reports including *Genetic Screening: ethical issues*.

Chapter 12

Successful marketing and public relations for your research project

No research project will ever succeed in enhancing knowledge or changing practice without successful marketing and PR. This chapter provides an introduction to the tools, tips and traps of marketing and PR.

Every day healthcare stories appear in newspapers, billboards, newsletters, on television, in magazines, on the radio, and, increasingly, on the Internet. The thirst for health information is ever present, but selective. Any PR exercise of your project has to compete with others trying to get their story out into a wider audience.

As to the 'audience', I use this term to cover a multitude of groups such as the potential and actual funders of your project, your managers, your peers, your host institution, professional groups and associations, voluntary agencies, advisory panels, patients, politicians, policy makers, the wider general public and the media.

But 'getting your story out' is not the first thing you should be thinking about when the letters 'PR' spring to mind. The first things to ask are 'why bother?' and 'what is the primary objective of a PR exercise for my research?'. Then you should ask 'can it be done?'. And from that you quickly get into questions such as who, what, where, how and when? If you have no, little or poor experience in PR then seek the counsel of some of those who have been involved in a PR health exercise.

Start thinking seriously about PR even before you have firmed up the project. Then you and your research team should become actively involved in PR exercises at every stage of the project (for the stages see the 'fate of research' pyramid, Chapter 8). Some of the best projects involve PR at every stage and keep a wide audience interested and informed on how the project is going. These have reached out to various audiences and interested parties and kept them informed of developments.

As an example, free-phone numbers can be established, and postage-paid postcards distributed. Newspaper, television and radio stories can feature the study; pharmacies and physician offices display study materials; public service announcements appear in local print and broadcast media. Experiences in these areas substantiate the need for a comprehensive co-ordinated approach, using planned multiple sources, to achieve success. Furthermore by engaging the lay and professional communities along with the media, costs can be kept to a minimum. They may also aid the inclusion of traditionally underserved groups of the population.

Various projects have also used different strategies and mediums of communication for different audiences and stages of work. The PR checklist shown in Box 12.1 will be useful to you and your research team.

The exact methods and time scales chosen for any PR exercise will depend on how the programme is run. PR is not a luxury: it is necessary to help a wider audience appreciate what you and your research team are doing and why.

PR can do many things, but it cannot:

- provide any guarantees of successful outcomes
- create stories out of thin-air
- control the media
- be done without time, money, people and resources being allocated to the exercise
- be easily, effectively and efficiently corrected if something goes wrong at any stage
- control all subsequent events, repercussions, and responses.

Box 12.1: Your public relations checklist

- Involve experts in PR early on in the programme – the organisation hosting the research may have its PR expert(s) but it always pays to think who is the best person/group for this piece of PR and speak to them.
- Be clear that 'news' is not treated the same way as 'features'.
- Assess what media is appropriate for your programme PR exercise (e.g. some have used features in women's magazines where the research programme involved breast cancer; some have used local schools where the issues were on alcoholism, smoking, paediatric care, obesity; another used local radio for a programme looking at care of the elderly living alone).
- Work in partnership with the PR experts to establish a coherent, cohesive strategy.

- Check you have permission/clearance from your research team, host organisation and sponsor to do the PR.
- Think about the implications and ramifications of the PR for your study subjects and those not in the study e.g. other patients.
- Decide in advance how you will record and measure the success of the PR exercise.
- Target audiences.
- Agree key messages.
- Agree who is giving out the messages (watch out, as this can become a very time-consuming activity in itself).
- Agree who else to inform about the story in advance of the media release/uptake.
- Provide points of contact for listeners/readers/media (name, position, telephone/fax/email details).
- Provide supporting material.
- Be aware that emotion and not reason may become involved as the PR unfolds.
- Be aware that your programme may upset others who are not being involved in their local research programme on the same issue.
- Do not do a PR exercise on the research programme unless you have programme members' approval.
- Be aware that the patients in the research study need to be in on the discussions before a PR exercise is carried out.
- Be aware that you lose control of the message once your story is out.
- Be aware that PR exercises can influence your programme.
- Be aware that good practice is to inform your whole organisation of the programme before going 'outside' with messages and stories.
- Review the exercise periodically with and without your PR expert input.
- If you are PRing at the start of the programme, PR also at the end.
- Remember PR is not just about promotion, it can affect many other areas of the programme such as recruitment, morale, and the dissemination of results.
- Before you do any PR, check with the funders of the programme and check with the ethics committee (this takes time so plan and discuss PR with these groups in advance – say what you plan to do, get approval and then do it).

Some of the worst examples of where PR went wrong is where it is done:

- without full and frank advanced consultation with all stakeholders in the research programme
- without a full and frank strategy for doing PR
- without considering in advance the implications of PR for the research programme and its members.

Although PR is increasingly being used in researchers' armamentarium, any PR exercise should not distract you or your team from the main business of your research programme.

Additional sources of help and advice

Below is a list of websites that will be of additional interest to you and your research team.

Department of Health

This site offers material produced by and for the Department of Health. Primarily used by health and social care professionals, academics and other interested parties, it is available for all parties to see. It includes press releases, and details of Department of Health publications, as well as information about the Department of Health, the NHS, and NHS Executive. www.doh.gov.uk

Department of Health Research and Development

This is the website for research and development (R&D) in the Department of Health. It includes details of the R&D Directorate, the Policy Research Programme, national R&D programmes as well as R&D in the regional offices. The National Research Register is also available on this site. www.doh.gov.uk/research

The Cochrane Collaboration

The Cochrane Collaboration is an international not-for-profit organisation. Its aim is to make up-to-date, accurate information about the effects of healthcare readily available worldwide. The major product of the collaboration is the Cochrane Database of Systematic Reviews

(CDSR) which is marketed as part of the Cochrane Library. Those who prepare the reviews are mostly healthcare professionals who volunteer to work in one of more than 40 collaborative review groups. Each review group has a co-ordinator, and an editorial team to oversee the quality of the group's reviews. The activities of the collaboration are directed by an elected steering group and are supported by staff in Cochrane centres around the world.

Cochrane Consumer Network

The Cochrane Consumer Network is part of the Cochrane Collaboration. It provides a co-ordinating network supporting consumers within Cochrane groups, as well as working to improve the quality of reviews, and make reviews more accessible to consumers. The network produces a newsletter that is available at www.cochraneconsumer.com.

The Cochrane Library

The Cochrane Library is an electronic publication designed to supply high-quality evidence to inform people providing and receiving healthcare, and those responsible for research, teaching, funding and administration at all levels. The Cochrane Library includes: CDSR, the Database of Abstracts of Reviews of Effectiveness (DARE) and the Cochrane Controlled Trials Register (CCTR). The abstracts of Cochrane reviews are available without charge on the Internet. www.cochrane.co.uk

INVOLVE (previously called The Consumer in NHS Research)

Based in Eastleigh near Southampton, INVOLVE support unit aims to:

- provide information, advice and support to consumers, researchers and those working in the NHS public health and social care on consumer involvement in research
- commission and undertake research about the involvement of consumers in such research

- produce publications and reports
- organise seminars, conferences and workshops on consumer involvement in health and social care research.

http://www.invo.org.uk

The NHS Centre for Reviews and Dissemination (CRD)

The NHS Centre for Reviews and Dissemination (CRD) was established in 1994 to provide the NHS with information on the effectiveness of treatments and the delivery and organisation of healthcare. The CRD undertakes and commissions credible, rigorous reviews of research findings on the effectiveness of healthcare relevant to the NHS. The CRD is also responsible for a series of reviews examining the effectiveness of health promotion interventions on behalf of the Health Education Authority. CRD disseminates the results of research to NHS decision makers. Within the NHS R&D programme, the CRD is the sibling organisation of the UK Cochrane Centre. CRD maintains databases of abstracts of good quality reviews of health research, abstracts of economic evaluations of health and health technology assessments. It also provides an information and enquiry service on reviews and economic evaluations for healthcare professionals, purchasers and providers, NHS managers, information providers, health service researchers and consumer organisations. www.york.ac.uk/inst/crd

The National Research Register

The National Research Register (NRR) is a register of ongoing and recently completed research projects funded by, or of interest to, the UK's National Health Service. The current release contains information on over 53 000 research projects, as well as entries from the Medical Research Council's Clinical Trials Register, and details on reviews in progress collected by the NHS CRD. www.doh.gov.uk/research/nrr.htm/

NHS Direct Online

This site provides information about healthy living and healthcare as well as a database of information for patients and the public on a variety of conditions. The database contains contact details for major national self-help groups and details of evaluated patient information leaflets and booklets on treatment choices. NHS Direct Online also contains a guide to the NHS. www.nhsdirect.nhs.uk

NHS R&D Health Technology Assessment (HTA) Programme

The HTA programme is a national programme of research established and funded by the Department of Health's R&D programme. The purpose of the programme is to ensure that high-quality research information on the costs, effectiveness and broader impact of health technologies is produced in the most effective way for those who use, manage and work in the NHS. The programme is overseen by the Standing Group on Health Technology (SGHT). The National Co-ordinating Centre for HTA (NCCHTA) which is part of the Wessex Institute for Health Research and Development at the University of Southampton, co-ordinates the HTA programme on behalf of the R&D programme. Every year the SGHT and its advisory panels, supported by the NCCHTA, decide which of the many suggestions received from the NHS and its users should become research priorities. The programme then issues calls for proposals, and commissions research to answer those questions. The results of the research are published as reports in the HTA monograph series. www.hta.nhsweb.nhs.uk

NHS R&D New and Emerging Applications of Technology (NEAT) Programme

The NEAT programme is one of three national NHS R&D programmes. The other two are the HTA and Service Delivery and Organisation (SDO) programmes. The current anticipated budget for NEAT is £5 million over five years. The main aim of NEAT is to promote and support, through applied research, the use of new or emerging technologies to develop healthcare products and interventions to enhance the quality, efficiency and effectiveness of health and social care. It will support strategic and applied research, the outputs of which must be generalisable and capable of being applied to a defined health or social care need. www.doh.gov.uk/research/rd3/nhsrandd

NHS R&D Service Delivery and Organisation (SDO) Programme

The SDO programme is one of three national NHS R&D programmes. The other two are the HTA and NEAT programmes. The programme director is Professor Sir John Pattison, Director of R&D. The aim of the programme is to produce and promote the use of research evidence about how the organisation and delivery of services can be improved to increase the quality of patient care, ensure better patient outcomes, and contribute to improved population health. The programme is being managed by a national co-ordinating centre (NCCSDO) at the London School of Hygiene and Tropical Medicine. The programme was formally launched in March 2000. A commissioning board to oversee the work and development of the programme has recently been established. The board membership comprises service users, healthcare professionals, health service managers, researchers and policy makers. www.sdo.lshtm.ac.uk

The metaRegister of Controlled Trials

The Current Controlled Trials metaRegister of Controlled Trials (mRCT) aims to promote the availability and exchange of information about randomised controlled trials in all areas of healthcare so that:

- researchers and funders can avoid duplicating research and wasting valuable resources
- reviews and meta-analysis can identify any possible publication bias
- patients and clinicians can have detailed and accurate information about therapies upon which to base their decisions.

The mRCT currently provides access to 15 major registers (about 6500 trial records) making it one of the largest controlled trials resources in the world. This is an excellent source of information for consumers wanting to become involved with RCTs. http://controlled-trials.com

Hub and Spokespeople

Alan Boyd of the Hub and Spokespeople project which is part of the Health for All Network is currently involved with some local level pilot projects to support consumer involvement in health service provision in general. This may be of interest to consumers involved in research. http://independent.livjm.ac.uk/healthforall/hubspoke/main.htm

Education for Participation

A course is being developed at Queen Margaret University, Edinburgh, designed to work with older people to enable them to feel more confident about participating in influencing the development of services. Using drama to explore how to make points in different ways; how to critically review documents; how to participate actively in meetings and to help older people express themselves. Each part of the course lasts 10 hours. For further details contact Belinda Dewar, Development and Research Manager, Scottish Centre for the Promotion of the Older Person's Agenda, Queen Margaret University, Edinburgh. Tel: 0131 317 3575 bdewar@qmuc.ac.uk

Strategies for Living

This is a project which has undertaken research involving mental health service users and has the following informative website: www.mentalhealth.org.uk.

Critical Appraisal Skills Programme (CASP)

The Critical Appraisal Skills Programme aims to 'enable decision makers and those who seek to influence them' to 'acquire skills and make sense of, and act on the evidence'. These workshops are likely to be useful for consumers wanting to become actively involved in research. http://www.phrw.org.uk

UK Co-ordinating Committee for Cancer Research (UKCCCR) Consumer Liaison Group

The Consumer Liaison Group was set up by the main committee of the UKCCCR in January 2000 following a period of consultation. There has been increasing recognition, over the past few years, of the need for consumer involvement across the whole framework of health services. http://ukcccr.icnet.uk/

Folk.us

Folk.us is a group of consumers and researchers in the south west who meet regularly in Exeter, run a training programme, and publish a newsletter. http://latis.ex.ac.uk/folk.us/findex.htm

Communitiesforhealth.net

This supports people in playing active roles in planning and implementing action. http://www.communitiesforhealth.net

Appendix 2

Contacts for various projects used in this text

Please note that due to the dynamic nature of people working in the NHS and academia, due to changes in NHS organisations' titles and telephone numbers, some of the details in the table below will naturally change over time. There should be enough detail in the table for you to get in touch with people behind each project. Otherwise try calling the organisations, try the additional sources of help and advice in Appendix 1or try web search engines.

Contacts for various projects used in this text

Title of topic	Contact details
Cancer voices	Ms Jane Bradburn, Project Manager, Cancerlink, 89 Albert Embankment, London SE1 7UQ. Tel: 020 7091 2013. Jane.bradburn@cancerlink.org.uk
Patient and carer views of stroke services	Ms Marcia Kelson, College of Health, 6 Spencer Gardens, London, SW14 7AH. Tel: 020 8392 1175. Marcia@tcoh.demon.co.uk
A randomised controlled trial to evaluate the benefit of a new information leaflet for parents of children hospitalised with benign febrile convulsions	Ms Fiona Paul, Lead Researcher, Tayside University Hospitals NHS Trust, Intensive Care Unit, Ninewells Hospital, Dundee, DD1 9SY. Tel: 01382 633820. Fiona.paul@tuht.scot.nhs.uk
A large randomised long-term assessment of the relative cost-effectiveness of surgery for Parkinson's disease	University of Birmingham Clinical Trials Unit, Park Grange, 1 Somerset Road, Edgbaston, Birmingham, B15 2RR. Tel: 0121 687 2314. Pd-trials@bham.ac.uk
Survey of views of people affected by motor neurone disease on the only drug treatment (then) available: riluzole	Ms Alison Morris, Co-ordinator, Motor Neurone Disease Association, PO Box 246, Northampton, NN1 2PR. Tel: 01604 611842. Alison.morris@mndassociation.org
Evaluating the multiple sclerosis (MS) specialist nurse: a review and development of the role	Ms Jane Johnson, Consultant Nurse – Neurorehabilitation, King's College Hospital NHS Trust, David Ferrier Ward, Ruskin Wing, King's College Hospital, Denmark Hill, London.

Title of topic	Contact details
Torbay Healthy Housing Group: Watcombe Project	Mr Andy Ruskin, Co-ordinator, RDSU, ITTC Building, Tamar Science Park, Plymouth, PL6 8BX. Tel: 01752 315112. Andrew.barton@phnt.swest.nhs.uk
Medication education	Professor Til Wykes, Project Leader, Institute of Psychiatry/SLAM NHS Trust, De Crespigny Park, London, SE5 8AF. Tel: 020 7848 0596. T.wykes@iop.kcl.ac.uk
Befriending: more than just finding friends?	Dr Carol Robinson, Lead Researcher, Norah Fry Research Centre, 3 Priory Road, Bristol, BS8 1TX. Tel: 0117 923 8137. C.e.robinson@bristol.ac.uk
Practice guidelines for primary healthcare teams to meet South Asian Carers' needs	Dr Savita Katbamna, Nuffield Community Care Studies Unit, University of Leicester, Department of Epidemiology and Public Health, 22–28 Princess Road West, Leicester, LE1 6TP. Tel: 0116 252 5439. Sk41@le.ac.uk
What happens to people with severe aphasia?	Dr Susie Parr, Department of Language and Communication Science, City University, London, EC1V 0HB. Tel: 0117 921 1192. susiepparr@btinternet.com
Collaborative studies on health service and quality of life in people with learning disability	Dr Sherva Cooray, Parkside Health Trust, Kingsbury Hospital, Honeypot Lane, London, NW9 9QY. Tel: 0208 451 8425. sherva.cooray@hertsmere-pct.nhs.uk
Joint replacement	Professor Paul Dieppe, Director, Medical Research Council Health Services Research Collaboration, Department of Social Medicine, University of Bristol, Canygne Hall, Whiteladies Road, Bristol, BS8 2PR. Tel: 0117 928 7343. P.dieppe@bristol.ac.uk
Cognitive remediation: a randomised controlled trial	Professor Til Wykes, Project Leader, Institute of Psychiatry/SLAM NHS Trust, De Crespigny Park, London, SE5 8AF. Tel: 020 7848 0596. T.wykes@iop.kcl.ac.uk
People's experiences of screening assessment by nurses in a community mental health team	Mr Martin Hird, Service User and Carer Co-ordinator, Leeds Community and Mental Health Trust, Tongue Lane, Leeds, LS6 4QB. Tel: 0113 295 2850. Martinhird-leedscmhst@hotmail.com
Disability equipment evaluations	Ms Helen Pain, Disability Equipment Assessment Centre, Southampton General Hospital, Level E, Centre Block 886, Tremona Road, Southampton, SO16 6YD. Tel: 023 8079 4576. Deac@soton.ac.uk
Cochrane skin group	Ms Colette Hoare, Recruitment of Consumers for Involvement in Research, National Eczema Society Skin Care Campaign, Hill House, Highgate Hill, London, N19 5NA. Tel: 020 7281 3553. choare@eczema.org
Developing and evaluating best practice for user involvement in cancer services	Mr James Rimmer, Project Manager, Avon, Somerset and Wiltshire Cancer Services, King's Square House, King's Square, Bristol, BS2 8EE. Tel: 0117 900 2323. james.rimmer@aswcs.nhs.uk

Index

accountability *27*, 67
   ethics committee 111
action research 92–5, *93*
   use in specific projects *78*, 95
advisory panels 44
advocacy groups 25, 28
age, factor in lay involvement 26
Alborz, A *et al.* 62–3
Allsop, J *et al.* 25
Andejeski, Y *et al.* 56
anonymity (participants) 88
aphasia research studies *5*
   benefits of lay involvement *23*
   lay participants *29*
   methods used *32*, *79*
   project contact details 138
   research design *78*
application procedures (ethics committee)
         114–18, *115*, *116*
   decision criteria 112–13, 116
   fees 114
   proposal rejections 116
   suitability of proposal 107–8, 110
assessment procedure evaluation studies *78*,
         79
   see also mental health service evaluations
The Association of Research Ethics
         Committees (AREC) 122
attitudes (research professionals) *15–16*, 45,
         49
audits, and ethic committee applications
         108

Bastian, H 60
befriending service evaluations
   benefits of lay involvement *23*
   lay participants *29*
   methods used *32*, *79*
   project contact details *138*
   research design *78*
benefits (lay involvement) *15*, 21–2, 57–8
   project-based evidence *23–4*
biomedical research *see* research programmes
Bogle, I 105
British Medical Association (BMA), Caldicott
         principles 103–5
BUPA Foundation 2

Caldicott Guardians 37, 103–5
   principles of good practice *104*
   website 105
cancer services evaluation projects *5*, *6*, 58–9,
         60
   benefits of lay involvement *23*, *24*
   Cancer Voices *5*, *137*
   lay participants *29*
   methods used *32–3*, *79*
   on nurse education studies 60
   research designs *78*
   UKCCCR Consumer Liaison Group 134–5
   on user involvement *6*, *138*
carers (South Asian) service evaluations *5*
   benefits of lay involvement *23*
   lay participants *29*
   methods used *32*, *79*
   project contact details *138*
   research design *78*
case studies, use in specific projects *78*
CASP *see* Critical Appraisal Skills Programme
CDMRP *see* Congressionally Directed medical
         research Programs
Central Office for Research Ethics Committee
         (COREC) 108, 121
Citizens Council 1–2
citizens' juries 71
Clayton, A *et al.* 30
Clift, R 70
clinical governance investigations, and ethics
         committee 108
clinical trial co-ordinating centres 53–4
clinical trials *see* research programmes
Clinical Trials Unit (Birmingham) 22
The Cochrane Collaboration 129–30
   Consumer Network 130
   Library 130
coercion 88
cognitive remediation evaluation *5*
   benefits of lay involvement *24*
   lay participants *29*
   methods used *33*, *79*
   project contact details 138
   research design *78*
cohort studies 81
   use in specific projects *78*, 81
commissions/rewards *16*

communication issues (research programmes) 50
see also public relations
communitiesforhealth.net 135
Community Health Councils (CHCs) 62–3
comparative studies, use in specific projects *78*
confidentiality 23, 36–7, 88, *98*
    Caldicott principles 103–5, *104*
    observational studies 80
Congressionally Directed medical research
    Programs (CDMRP) 22
consensus conferences 72–3
    costs 71
consent (patient) 63
    and interviews *90*
consultations
    at local level 34, 60, 69–70
    at national level 68–9
    PCG/Ts and local communities 62–3
    People's Panel 70
consumer advocates, as lay representatives
    25
consumer involvement *see* lay involvement
The Consumer in NHS Research (INVOLVE)
    130–1
Convention on Human Rights and
    Biomedicine (Council of Europe)
    122–3
Conway, G 74
cost-effectiveness studies *see* Parkinson's
    disease treatment evaluations
costs
    of citizens' jury 71
    participant's expenses 35
    of polls 70
    see also resource allocation
CRD *see* The NHS Centre for Reviews and
    Dissemination
Critical Appraisal Skills Programme (CASP)
    134
cross-over trials, use in specific projects *79*

Daniels, J 22
Danish Board of Technology, consensus
    conferences 72–3
data collection
    legislation 37, 103, 123
    methods *78*, *79*
    planning considerations *98*
Data Protection Act 37, 103, 123
Davies, C 26–8, *27*
Declaration of Helinski 37, 122
deliberative polling 70
Delphi technique 85–7
Department of Health
    Caldicott report and related guidance 123

Convention on Human Rights and
    Biomedicine draft additional protocols
    123
    website 129
Department of Health Research and
    Development 129
Department of Health and Social Care
    Research and Development Office 2
diabetes service evaluations, South Asian
    women's group 57–8
disability equipment evaluations *6*
    benefits of lay involvement *24*
    lay participants *29*
    methods used *33*, *79*
    project contact details 138
    research design *78*
Dixon, P *et al.* 43
documentary analysis 77–80
    use in specific projects *79*
Doll, R 81

Earl-Slater, A 77, 92
e-mail surveys, Delphi techniques 86
effectiveness (lay involvement), PCG/Ts and
    local communities 61–3
Ely, JW *et al.* 81
employment, factor in lay involvement 26
Entwhistle, V *et al.* 43
Environment Council, Brent Spar disposal 73
ethical issues 88
    Citizens Council recommendations 1–2
    human rights 121–3
    in observational studies 80
    see also confidentiality
ethics committees 107–18
    application decisions 112, 116
    conditions of approval 112–13
    lay involvement in trial applications 121
    local research ethics committees (LRECs)
        107–8, 114–16
    multicentre research ethics committees
        (MRECs) 109–18
    proposal suitability criteria 107–8, 110
    structure and procedure guidance 121–2
ethnic minority user groups
    and lay involvement 57–8
    see also carers (South Asian) service
        evaluations
ethnographic evidence studies
    use in specific projects *5*, *78*, *79*
    see also aphasia research
European Union, Convention on Human
    Rights and Biomedicine 122–3
evaluation/monitoring
    and ethics committees 118
    of lay involvement *6*, 48–9, 118

evaluation studies *78*
    see also cancer services evaluation projects
Evans, J 81

facilitators
    and ethnic user groups 57
    role in focus groups 84
'fate of clinical research' pyramid 97–100, *99*
febrile convulsions service evaluation *5*
    benefits of parental involvement *23*
    lay participants *29*
    methods used *32, 79*
    research design *78*
feedback (participant) 48–9, *89*
    and action research 94
Fisher, F 105
Flanagan, J 60
focus groups 70–1, 83–5
    use in specific projects *34, 79*
Folk.us 135
follow-up *see* evaluation/monitoring
foresight programmes 70–1
frameworks *see* strategies
Frater, A 26
Freemantle, N *et al.* 82
The Freedom of Information Act (2000) 123
funding
    BUPA Foundation 2
    DoH and Social Care Research and
        Development Office 2
    NEAT programmes 132

gender, factor in lay involvement 26
gene therapy research, Wellcome Trust 70
The General Medical Council, Standards of
        Practice 123
genetic testing, and citizens' juries 71
genetically modified (GM) crop research,
        consensus conferences 73
Glasgow, RE *et al.* 81
government policy
    public engagement 67–8
    see also Department of Health
Graham, J *et al.* 59
Grant-Pearce, C *et al.* 26
group dynamics, effects on research trials 84,
        85
group representatives 60

Hampshire County Council, waste
        management consultations 69–70
*The Handbook of Clinical Trials and Other
        Research* 77
Hanley, B *et al.* 14–16, *15, 16,* 43, 53–4
Health for All Network 133–4

health authorities, as programme hosts/
        sponsors 51–2
health committees, and lay involvement 61
health information services, and needs-led
        research 54
health professionals
    as lay representatives 25–6
    regulation and lay involvement 26–8, *27*
    and research projects *see* research
        professionals
health promotion, and advisory group work 58
Heller, T *et al.* 55–6
Hogg, C 61
host organisations 51, *99*
    commitment *51*
    strategies for lay involvement *51–2*
    see also sponsors
Hub and Spokespeople project (Health for All)
        133–4
human genome mapping, consensus
        conference (Denmark) 73
The Human Rights Act (1998) 122
human rights guidance 122–3

Independent Complaints Advocacy Service
        (ICAS) 68
information and advice sources (lay
        involvement) 129–35, 137–8
    recruitment 28, 33–4
information sharing
    advisory group work 58
    see also confidentiality
inspections, and lay involvement 71–2
internet dialogues 74
interviews 87–9
    possible problems *90*
    practical considerations 88–9
    use in specific projects *79*
INVOLVE (The Consumer in NHS Research)
        130–1
*Involving Patients and the Public in
        Healthcare* (DoH 2001) 67–8
irradiated food acceptability studies 72–3

joint replacement treatment evaluations *6*
    benefits of lay involvement *24*
    lay participants *29*
    methods used *33, 79*
    project contact details 138
    research design *78*

Kelson, M 26
Klein, AR *et al.* 60

lay involvement
    barriers *see* participation problems

benefits and rationale *15*, 21–2, *23–4*,
57–8
confidentiality 23, 36–7, 80, 88, 98, 103–5
v. 'consumer' involvement 4–6
defined 3–4
effectiveness promotion 58–9, 60
equality of access 45
evaluation of involvement 6, 48–9, 118
factors affecting involvement 44–6, *45–6*,
48, *98–9*
host commitment *51–2*
information advice sources 129–35, *137–8*
legal position 37–8, 121–3
objectives 28, 46–7, 49
participant motivations 24, 48
payments 34–6, 72, 88
planning consideration checklist *98–9*
programme types *see* lay involvement
projects
representativeness 14, 25–8
selection of participants *27, 28, 29, 30,
31–4*
stages/processes 31–4, *31, 32–3*
strategies 30–1, 43–52, 79
timing 31
training issues *see* training
see also participants
lay involvement projects *5–6*
citizens' juries 71
clinical trial co-ordinating centres 53–4
consensus conferences 72–3
consultations at local level 62–3, 69–70
consultations at national level 67, 68–9
deliberative polling 70
focus groups 70–1
foresight programmes 75
health committees/councils 61–3
inspections 71–2
internet dialogues 74
multicentre research ethics committees
(MRECs) *116*
and needs-led research 54–5
primary care groups/trusts (PCG/Ts) 61–3
self-assessments 61–2
stakeholder dialogues 73–4
standing consultative panels 70
Trust boards 61–3
see also specific projects
leadership 49
learning disabilities service evaluations
(quality of life) 5
contact details *138*
lay participants *29*
and meaningful participation 55–6
methods used *33*, 79
research design 78

legal issues 37–8
ethics committee recommendations 108
planning considerations *99*
literature searches, use in group decision
making 60
Local Authority Overview and Scrutiny Clinics
(LAOSC) 68
local research ethics committees (LRECs)
107–8, 114–16
application suitability 107–8, 116
Central Office for Research Ethics
Committees website 108
links with MRECs 14–16, *115*
Local Voices (NHS Executive 1992) 21

Macara, S 105
Market and Opinion Research International
(MORI) 70
market research
citizens' juries 71
focus groups 70–1
People's Panel 70
marketing research projects 50, 125–8
checklist *126–7*
media involvement 125–8, *126–7*
The Medical Research Council (MRC) 2, 123
medication education research 5
benefits of lay involvement 23
lay participants *29*
methods used *32*, 79
project contact details *138*
research design 78
mental health service evaluations 6, 55
benefits of lay involvement *24*, 55
lay participants *29*
methods used *33*, 79
project contact details *138*
research design 78
Strategies for Living project 134
The metaRegister of Controlled Trials (mRCT)
133
Monsanto, and stakeholder dialogues 74
Montgomery, A and Fahey, T 14, 17
MORI *see* Market and Opinion Research
International
motivational factors (participants) 24, 48
and recognition programmes 48
motor neurone treatment evaluations 5
benefits of lay involvement 23
lay participants *29*
methods used *32*, 79
project contact details *137*
research design 78
Muhib, F *et al.* 34
multicentre research ethics committees
(MRECs) 109–18

cross-referrals 113
decision criteria 112–13
lay involvement *116*
legal liability 110–11
links with local centres 114–16, *115*
membership 110, *116*
procedural flowchart *115*
progress reports 116–18, *117*
multiple sclerosis service evaluations 5
benefits of lay involvement *23*
lay participants *29*
methods used *32*, 79
project contact details 137
research design *78*

National Co-ordinating Centre for Health
Technology Assessment (NCCHTA)
55, 132
National Institute for Clinical Excellence
(NICE), Citizens Council 1–2
The National Research Register (NRR) 131
National Tracker Survey 62
NCCHTA *see* NHS Research and
Development (R&D) programmes
NEAT *see* NHS Research and Development
(R&D) programmes
needs-led research 54–5
The New NHS (DoH 1995) 21
The NHS Centre for Reviews and
Dissemination (CRD) 131
NHS Direct Online 131–2
NHS information strategy 103–5
NHS Research and Development (R&D)
programmes 132–3
Health Technology Assessment Programme
(NCCHTA) 132
New and Emerging Applications of
Technology (NEAT) 132
Service Delivery and Organisation (SDO)
133
non-probability sampling 34
Nuffield Council on Bioethics 123

objectives (research programmes) 28, 46–7, 49
SMART 50
observational studies 80–1
use in specific projects 79
see also cohort studies
Ochocka, J *et al.* 55
Oliver, S 53, 54–5
organisational strategies *51–2*
outcome measures, use in specific projects
79

Parkinson's disease treatment evaluations
benefits of Society's involvement 22, *23*

lay participants *29*
methods used *32*, 79
project contact details 137
research design *78*
participants
and age 26
attitude studies 22
choice and selection issues 3–6, *27*, 28, *29*,
30, 31–4
with cognitive impairments 55–6
information sources for 28, 33–4
involvement considerations *98–9*
legal status 37–8, 121–3
motivational factors 24, 48
payment considerations 34–6, 72, 88
representativeness 13–14, 25–8, 55–6
screening 47
social/educational class 26–7
viewpoint and perspective 13–14, *16*
participation problems 53
attitudes of research professionals *45–6*
cognitive impairment 55–6
conflicting viewpoints 16, *16*
lack of resources 59
language differences 55, 57
loss of confidence *45–6*, 74
self-selection 74
Patient Advocacy and Liaison Services (PALS)
68
and research 68
Patient Forums 68
payment considerations 34–6, 72, 88
peer support 60
People's Panel 70
perspectives
analytical *14*
participant 13–16
v. representativeness 13–14, 25–8
pilot studies 80
questionnaires 89
planning considerations *90*, *98–9*
see also research methods
postal surveys
Delphi techniques 86
primary care and lay involvement feedback
61–2
pressure groups, lay involvement 28
primary care groups/trusts (PCG/Ts) 61–2
local consultations 62–3
progress reports *115*, 116
prospective/future predictive investigations
cohort studies 81
foresight programmes 70–1
public consultation *see* consultations
public relations 48, 50, 125–8
checklist *126–7*

qualitative research
  People's Panel 70
  use in specific projects *78*
  see also Delphi techniques
quantitative research, People's Panel 70
Queen Margaret University (Edinburgh),
     educating older participants 134
questionnaires 89–92
  question types/techniques *91–2*
  use in specific projects *79*
questions for research programme planners 90,
    98–9

random sampling 34
randomised controlled trials 82
  clinical trial co-ordinating centres study
    14–16, *15, 16*
  use in specific projects *78*, 82
recognition programmes 48
record keeping 49, *117*
recruitment *15*, 47, 49
reflective approaches, needs-led research 54
Reid, S *et al.* 81
representativeness 13–14, 25–8
  and meaningful participation 55–6
research methods 77–95
  action research 92–5
  cohort study 78, 81
  Delphi technique 85–7
  documentary analysis 77–80
  focus group 83–5
  interviews 87–9
  observational study 80–1
  questionnaires 89–92
  randomised controlled trials 14–16, *15, 16*,
    78, 82
  systematic review 82–3
research professionals 49
  attitudes *15, 16*, 45–6
  leadership 49
research programmes
  application procedures 107, 112–18, *115,
    116, 117*
  evaluations 118
  failures/rejections 100, 112, 116
  information advice sources 122, 129–35,
    137–8
  management *45*, 47–9
  marketing and public relations 48, 125–8,
    126–7
  objectives 28, 46–7, 49–50
  planning consideration checklist *98–9*
  project design 47, *51*, 78
    see also research methods
  Public Consultation workshops 69
  pyramid model 97–100, *99*

record keeping 49, *117*
register of projects 131
resource allocation 35, 45, 59
rights and obligations websites 122
sponsors *see* host organisations
stages/processes 31–4, *31, 32–3, 99*, 100,
    115
  see also ethical issues; lay involvement
    projects
resource allocation 46, 59
  participant's expenses 35
retrospective investigations, cohort studies 81
Rhodes, P *et al.* 56–7, *57–8*
Rowe, R 61–2

sampling methods 34
satisfaction surveys, People's Panel 70
scientific review panels, consumer
    involvement 56
SDO *see* NHS Research and Development
    (R&D) programmes
Select Committee on Science and Technology
  irradiated food acceptability 73
  public engagement methods 67
self-help groups
  and lay involvement *29*
  needs-led research 54
Service Delivery and Organisation (SDO) 133
service users, as lay members *29*
service users' advisory groups 56–7
Simeonsson, RJ *et al.* 13–14
skin disorder review studies 6
  benefits of lay involvement *24*
  lay participants *29*
  methods used *33*, 79
  project contact details 138
  research design 78
SMART objectives 50
Smith, C and Armstrong, D 26
Smith, SL *et al.* 34
social class, factor in lay involvement 26, *27*
Social Services Inspectorate (SSI), volunteer
    inspectors 71–2
sponsors
  ethics committee application fees
    (commercial companies) 114
  influence 89
  queries *99*
  see also host organisations
stakeholder dialogues 73–4
standing consultative panels 70
Stevens, T *et al.* 58–9
strategies 30–1, 43–52, *44*
  factors affecting involvement 44–6, *45–6*
Strategies for Living project 134
stroke service evaluations 5

benefits of lay involvement 23
lay participants 29
methods used 32, 79
project contact details 137
research design 78
studies of views/experiences 78
systematic review, use in specific projects 78, 82–3

telephone surveys, Delphi technique 86
Telford, R *et al.* 4–6
time-space sampling (TSS) 34
Torbay Healthy Housing Group: Watcombe Project *see* Watcombe Project
training (participants) 47–8, 49, 55
    Critical Appraisal Skills Programme (CASP) 134
    DoH and Social Care Research and Development Office funding 2
    Folk.us 135
    Queen Margaret University (Edinburgh) 134
training (professionals), influence of lay participants 59–60
treatment options, lay perspectives 13–14
trust, public v. decision takers 70

UK Co-ordinating Committee for Cancer Research (UKCCCR), Consumer Liaison Group 134–5

USA experiences 22
user groups, and lay involvement 29

value systems 46
    research processes 55
venue-based time-space sampling 34
voluntary organisations, and lay involvement 29
volunteer inspectors, SSI recruitment and training programme 71–2

Walshe, K *et al.* 50
Watcombe Project (Torbay) 5, 138
    lay participants 29
    methods used 32, 78
    project contact details 138
    project design 79
Wellcome Trust, gene therapy research 70
Wellwood, J *et al.* 13
Welsh Institute for Health and Social Care, genetic testing 71
Williamson, C 26, 61
Willison, DJ *et al.* 63
Wilson-Barnett, J 59–60
Wood, J 59–60
World Health Organization (WHO), guidelines for ethics committees website 122
The World Medical Association (WMA), Declaration of Helinski 122